Your INSIDE GUIDE to the

EMERGENCY DEPARTMENT

And How to Prevent Having to Go!

Dr. Fred Voon
MD, CCFP-EM

◆ FriesenPress

Suite 300 - 990 Fort St
Victoria, BC, V8V 3K2
Canada

www.friesenpress.com

Visit www.DrVoon.com for Internet links and downloadable forms you can use and share.

Books and e-books, excerpts and e-excerpts, are available for bulk sales and quantity discounts.

E-mail me at book@drvoon.com for more information or licensing opportunities.

ISBN
978-1-77760-341-0 (Hardcover)
978-1-77760-340-3 (Paperback)
978-1-77760-342-7 (eBook)

1. HEALTH & FITNESS, HEALTH CARE ISSUES
2. HEALTH & FITNESS, DISEASES
3. HEALTH & FITNESS, FIRST AID

Distributed to the trade by The Ingram Book Company

PRAISE FOR YOUR INSIDE GUIDE TO THE EMERGENCY DEPARTMENT

"A great read. Wish everyone could read this before coming to the ER."

Dianne Walter, Emergency RN

"An insider's guide on how the ER works, who should go, and maybe who does not need to. This is packed together with a bunch of simple advice on how to take care of common health problems. A fascinating read."

Dr. James Heilman
Emergency Physician, Wikipedia Editor, Wikimedia Foundation Trustee

"Well written, easy to follow & read, clear and concise. Intriguing, interesting, practical & useful information. Would make a great household book."

Laureen Bali, Emergency RN

"This is a thoughtful resource, offering exceptional insights into the emergency department and helping the public make informed decisions about their visit. This guide truly illustrates the UBC Faculty of Medicine's deep commitment and contract with society, placing the patient and public at the centre of everything we do."

Dr. Dermot Kelleher
MB, MD, FRCP, FRCPI, FMedSci, FCAHS, FRCPC, AGAF
Dean, Faculty of Medicine Vice-President, Health
The University of British Columbia

"Dr. Voon has written a book that is much needed. He has demystified, with relevant information and in clear language, what is happening in Emergency Rooms that should calm those who read it and then feel the need to visit an ER. And isn't that most of us at some point? Anything that can be done to lessen the high anxiety and worry that everyone will have when they feel they need that kind of help is to be applauded. Dr. Voon's motivation in writing this book is clear: he wishes to improve the patient experience when dealing with the health care system. That should tell you lots about what kind of physician he is."

Bruce Wright, MD, CCFP, FCFP
Regional Associate Dean, Vancouver Island

Faculty of Medicine, University of British Columbia
Head, Division of Medical Sciences
University of Victoria

AUTHOR'S NOTE, DISCLAIMER, AND DISCLOSURE

This book is not intended as a substitute for the medical attention, advice, examination, or treatment delivered by a physician. The reader should consult a healthcare professional for all matters relating to health, particularly issues that may require diagnosis or medical attention.

Even if the information in this book suggests medical attention is not needed, readers who think they have an emergency medical concern can and should go to their nearest Emergency Department (ED) or call an ambulance. **If in doubt, get checked out!**

This book provides—by necessity—only general information. It cannot and does not take into account individuals' health statuses and their various medical, physical, or emotional situations and needs. Even in person, physicians are always weighing risks versus benefits to the individual patient in front of them—so there is truly no "one size fits all" approach to emergency medicine.

Also, be aware that what doctors believe to be true changes with time and with newer evidence. The information in this book is only current to the date of publication and medical opinions could change in the future. When I teach medical students I say, "today's gospel is tomorrow's mythology" because some of the beliefs that were current in my early career have shifted or even been reversed. However, most of what I have chosen to write about in this book hasn't changed since I started medical school 20 years ago.

I do not have a financial interest in any of the products I mention in this book. I am not affiliated with, and this book is not endorsed by, any of the companies who manufacture the products mentioned. I do not receive any money for prescribing medications (generic or branded) or ordering tests or referring people to other healthcare providers. My income does not go up or down based on how many patients present to the ED. If anything, I am motivated to keep those patients who don't really need to be there out of the ED in order to free up resources for the critically ill and injured.

DEDICATION

To my father for his gift of adaptability
To my mother for her gift of devotion
To my brother for his enthusiasm
To my sister for her creativity
To my kids for their resilience

TABLE OF CONTENTS

PREFACE xiii

PART 1: THINKING OF GOING TO THE EMERGENCY DEPARTMENT? 1

You've Decided You Need to Go to the ED 3

Do Not Call Ahead 3

What and Whom Should You Bring? 4

What Happens in the ED? 8

Triage 8

Registration 9

Waiting 10

Nurse Assessment 11

Physician Assessment 14

Investigations 15

Treatment 17

Discharge 21

Admission 22

What Is the Emergency Department NOT Good At? 24

What are Emergency Personnel Not Good At? 27

PART 2: HURRY UP… AND WAIT 29

Why Are You Waiting So Long? 31

Why Did That Other Person Get Called Before You? 34

How to Speed Up Your Visit and Streamline Your Care 37

What If You Are Not Sure About Whether You Should Go to the ED? 40

Is There a Good Time of Day to Visit So You Wait Less? 43

Why Can't You Lie Down Somewhere? Can You Stay in a Stretcher? 44

Why Do You Have to Tell Your Story Again and Again? 46

PART 3: PEOPLE AND PLACES   **47**

Why I Love Being an Emergency Physician   49

Who Are All These People?   50

Basic Emergency Department Layout   54

PART 4: ARMCHAIR EMERG DOC   **57**

The Internet Will See You Now   59

Time-sensitive Conditions   60

Worrisome to Patients, But Not an Emergency After All   64

Your Symptoms and What They Might Mean   68

     Pain   *69*

     Fever   *70*

Home Medicine Cabinet   72

What Doesn't Work?   79

The Life of a Typical Viral Infection   81

Tips and Tricks for Common Conditions   83

     Allergic Reaction   *83*

     Back Pain   *85*

     Concussion   *90*

     Eczema   *92*

     Fainting   *92*

     Gastroenteritis, a.k.a. "Stomach Flu"   *95*

     Mild Burns   *98*

     Nasal Congestion   *99*

     Nosebleeds   *101*

     Skin Infections   *102*

     Swallowing Stuff   *104*

     Wounds and Wound Care   *104*

Not So Common… But May Save You a Trip to the Emergency   109

     Bruising Under a Fingernail or Toenail   *109*

     Nursemaid's Elbow ("pulled elbow" or radial head subluxation)   *110*

     Something Up the Nose   *112*

     Vertigo (benign paroxysmal positional vertigo, BPPV)   *113*

APPENDICES   **115**

   Appendix 1. ABCs of Prevention   117

   Appendix 2. Internet Sites I Trust   122

   Appendix 3. Sample Medical History Summary   125

   Appendix 4. Advance Directive   127

   Appendix 5. What Changes During a Pandemic?   130

   Appendix 6. Glossary   133

   Appendix 7. List of Side Bars   137

REFERENCES   **139**

ACKNOWLEDGMENTS   **141**

ABOUT THE AUTHOR   **143**

BULK SALES   **145**

PREFACE

The Emergency Department (ED) is a critical part of our healthcare system. We are open 24 hours a day. We never close and, in Canada, we never turn people away. The ED is there for people who can't see their regular doctor, and who have medical emergencies and need immediate, often life-saving, treatment. We also prepare for mass casualty situations such as natural disasters or industrial accidents.

As a physician trained in Family Medicine and Emergency Medicine in Canada, I have seen many different systems for urgent and acute care. Of course, I've also ended up on the other side of the stretcher when I've brought family members to the ED. While I am writing from the context of a typical Canadian hospital, much of what I describe may be applicable in other settings as well. A few methods vary by city and country, but there are many things that seem to be common to different places I've worked (Alberta, British Columbia, New Brunswick, Nova Scotia, and even New Zealand). Practice patterns and terminology may vary in the USA or abroad, or in rural and remote communities, but there are probably more similarities than differences. While each hospital may have their own particular systems, a similar approach to emergency medicine is used around the globe. The Emergency Department may be called the Accident and Emergency Department, the Urgent Care Department, or the Emergency Room. In this book, I will refer to it as the ED.

When pain or illness strikes, heading straight to the local ED can seem like the right thing to do. My colleagues and I are, however, occasionally amazed at what people have or haven't done prior to coming to the hospital, and their reasons for it. ED doctors and nurses are sometimes *not* the most appropriate healthcare professionals to be dealing with your condition. You may be in for a long wait to be seen, only to eventually be given treatments that you could have bought over-the-counter at your local pharmacy. Perhaps you may be better off trying your primary care provider or a walk-in clinic.

It can certainly be confusing to navigate the healthcare system, and we as health professionals have not done the best job educating the public about how best to use and access the system, and what to expect. Patients repeatedly have misunderstandings and misconceptions about what happens in the ED, leaving people frustrated and wondering why it can take four (or more) hours to finally see a doctor.

This book offers a guided tour of a standard ED and an introduction to the team of healthcare professionals who look after thousands of Canadians every day. My aim is to give you insights into what we do in the ED, how things work, when to go and when to stay at home, how to speed up your visit, and the importance of following the advice you are given when you leave the ED. I also put forward an assortment of reminders of how a little prevention goes a long way, and where common-sense precautions can dramatically reduce the risk of serious illness or injury. Hopefully, much of the information in this book will help you make more informed choices for yourself and your loved ones.

This book is not for everyone!

Some people need specific attention and should not hesitate to go to the ED if they are worried about something.

These include but are not limited to:

- Pregnant women

- Infants and young children

- People with chronic and serious medical conditions such as kidney disease, liver disease, heart failure, or a compromised immune system

- Any person who is taking many medications (because of risk of interactions)

Call 9-1-1 for:

- Any person who has been badly injured or burned

- Any person who is having signs of heart attack or stroke

- Any person who is having trouble breathing

- Severe allergic reactions

Remember, if you are worried and in doubt about whether you need to call 9-1-1 for a medical emergency, call.

PART 1
THINKING OF GOING TO THE EMERGENCY DEPARTMENT?

You've Decided You Need to Go to the ED

If you are heading to the ED, chances are you are injured, in pain, or feeling really sick with symptoms that aren't familiar. It is reasonable to feel nervous wondering what the root cause is, or anxious about what tests or procedures you might need. You could also be distressed because your regular doctor, who knows you well, isn't available. The ED is there for just these circumstances, but it can seem like an intimidating and chaotic place with doctors, nurses, paramedics, and patients in all directions. However, there actually is a structure and logic to what is going on, and as part of your "Inside Guide to the ED," I am going to explain how this very important part of our healthcare system works.

Do Not Call Ahead

If you are uncertain about going to your local ED it might be tempting to call and find out what the wait time is. **Please don't!**

- The person who answers will probably be a clerk, not a medical professional, and will not be able to give you a specific answer. They will also not be able to provide any medical advice.
- The ED doesn't take reservations like a restaurant.
- The situation can change in a flash. Even if it's taking two hours to see a doctor when you call, by the time you arrive the wait could be one hour or five hours.

Please note that due to privacy and confidentiality, the ED staff cannot provide detailed information about patients, even if they are your loved one, over the phone. We also have no way to know for certain who is calling.

> "If you are going to base your decision around how long the wait is, the chances are the emergency department isn't the right place for you"
>
> – Juliette Hughes, Southmead Hospital

MYTH: If I call 9-1-1 and go to the ED by ambulance, I will be seen faster by a doctor.

FACT: Ambulances are available for emergencies. When you call 9-1-1, paramedics arrive to help. They can diagnose some conditions, give certain medications and do some interventions. If necessary, they will communicate with the ED about your situation. However, you won't necessarily get seen by the ED doctor any sooner than if you'd been dropped off by a taxi or neighbour. You will go through the exact same triage process as all patients. And don't forget that you will also be sent a bill for the ambulance and paramedic service.

There are a limited number of ambulances in any region, and if one is being used for a patient with a non-urgent issue, then there are fewer ambulances available in the event of a real emergency like a cardiac arrest that happens at the swimming pool, or a major collision on the highway.

BUT ... there are circumstances when calling 9-1-1 is essential! Paramedics who arrive on the scene can regularly deliver life-saving treatments on the way to the ED. Call 9-1-1 immediately if you suspect a heart attack or stroke, or for a serious accident, choking, major burns, severe allergic reactions, or drowning. If you are unsure if it's a medical emergency, and are worried it could be, it is better to call 9-1-1.

What and Whom Should You Bring?

One of the most helpful things you can bring is an advocate. This could be a family member, friend, co-worker, neighbour, or care aide. They can be there to help find you a blanket if you're feeling cold, signal the nurse if your symptoms are getting worse, or listen for your name to be called (especially if you have to use the washroom or pay for parking). Don't worry if aspects of your health concern are personal or confidential—you can always ask your advocate to leave when the doctors and nurses talk to you and examine you. However, if you trust them to be present for those interactions, they might remember things that you might miss. Although I try to give resources or written discharge instructions to most of my patients, information from healthcare personnel can be forgotten or misunderstood. When you're not at your best and the healthcare team members are pressed for time, it can be a recipe for errors. Having someone with a clear head with you (even if they are also concerned about your health) can reduce miscommunication and misunderstandings. If you can not bring another person with you, bring a pen and paper to write down key information given to you or that you want to pass along.

To assist your healthcare team and reduce the hardship of waiting, here are a few suggestions of things to bring (and not bring). Consider having some of these things ready to go in case of a health emergency.

Do bring

- Your provincial health card.
- A list of your current medications, including over-the-counter medications, herbals, or other "natural" products. Note any recent changes to medications.
- A list of your medical conditions and previous surgeries. You may be asked about these multiple times by different people. (See Appendix 3 for a sample of a medical history summary you may wish to complete and carry with you.)
- A small notepad and pen
- Your medications so you don't miss a dose. We may only have basic medications.
- Earplugs. It can get quite noisy at times.
- Your walker or wheelchair, if you use one.
- Something to read.
- Your glasses or hearing aids so you can understand, plus whatever you store them in.
- Something to watch or listen to on your phone or tablet, using earbuds so you don't disturb others in the waiting room. (Please remember, however, that there may not be Wi-Fi or a place to charge your electronics.)
- Comfortable clothing that, ideally, is easy to put on and take off quickly.
- Some cash or a credit card for parking, food and beverage outlets, or vending machines.

- Optional: A small water bottle and snack, especially if you have diabetes or have food restrictions. (Do check with your nurse first, however, as we prefer that patients keep an empty stomach for certain medical reasons.)

Don't bring

- A lot of people. There is generally not enough space, and the ED waiting room is not a pleasant place to spend time.
- Strong scents or food. Many people are sensitive to scents such as perfumes. The person waiting beside you may have nausea or a migraine that could be worsened by certain smells.
- Lots of layers of clothing and accessories. We have to examine patients at skin level, and it can be hard to do a complete exam with bulky clothing in the way.
- Valuables, jewelry, suitcases, or large backpacks/duffle bags. You may be moved through multiple locations, with little room for personal belongings, and no secure storage.
- Flammables, weapons, needles, drugs, or alcohol. This should be pretty obvious.

Planning to Go? Plan to Come Back!

Often, our nurses have to hold discharged patients because there are barriers to getting home safely, which creates delays in caring for other patients. Spend a couple of minutes thinking about how you are going to get back home (especially if you are arriving by ambulance, or in the middle of the night).

- Bring your house keys. If you are locked out of your building, will you be able to get back in?
- Whom can you call upon if you need a ride? Do you have their phone number?
- Don't forget footwear if you come by ambulance. Nurses tell me they periodically have to send people home in socks or disposable booties!

Sometimes patients are unable to safely drive after their ED visit, for example after dilating eye drops for examination, opioids for pain or sedation, or a cast on the leg or arm. If you drive, what would happen if you had to leave your car in the parking lot?

What Happens in the ED?

Triage

No matter how you arrive–whether on foot, by ambulance, or sent in by another doctor—your first stop will be at the Triage Desk. Here a nurse will ask you a few basic questions (such as your age and why you came to the ED) and check your vital signs (such as your temperature, heart rate, and blood pressure). This information helps the Triage Nurse determine how serious your condition is or might become. The ED uses a triage category system that indicates how urgently a patient needs to be seen. In the USA, the scale ranks patients from 1 to 5 with 1 being the most urgent. In Canada, colours correspond to each level. The triage category is added to your particular file, but this information is not shared with patients. Rather it is used to help the ED staff decide whom to see when. The table below explains the categories in each country.

American and Canadian Triage Category Systems

USA Emergency Severity Index (ESI)	Meaning (from most serious to least serious)	Canada Canadian Triage and Acuity Scale (CTAS)
1	Resuscitation	Blue
2	Emergent	Red
3	Urgent	Yellow
4	Less Urgent	Green
5	Non-Urgent	Grey/White

Registration

All patients need to be registered. After triage, you will be sent to another desk where a clerk will ask for your name, date of birth, address and phone numbers, your health card number and any insurance information, and emergency contact information. Make sure all this information is correct so that we can contact you or someone you trust. The clerk will also ask you the name of your family physician/general practitioner (FP/GP) or primary care provider (PCP) if you have one. This is important because we will then send them a report about your visit, test results, and recommended follow-up after you leave the ED. (Next time you see your usual doctor, be sure to mention your visit to the ED so that he or she can look for this correspondence in your chart.)

The registration clerk enters your information into the ED's computer system. The system keeps track of who is waiting to be seen, where they are located (for instance in the waiting room or a special examination room), and what tests might be pending or completed. The system also creates an encounter or "chart" that ED staff use to document more of your medical history and past surgeries or treatments, to order lab work (like blood or urine tests) or imaging (like X-rays), and to record diagnoses. If you have ever been a patient in that hospital, they can also find your records from your previous visits there.

Electronic Health Records

MYTH: All your health information is kept up to date in one central place and shared between all your doctors.

FACT: With modern technology, it's easier to make and store digital copies of patient reports, notes, and referrals. However, there are many different electronic health record systems in use that don't connect or "talk" to each other. If your medical visits are within the same hospital or region, your records may be quite complete and in one place. But that may not be the case if you're from out of town or even if you visit different hospitals and clinics in the same city. This includes your medication profile. Some systems can access what you are taking through pharmacy records but others are unable to determine what you are taking accurately.

Waiting

You may find you are waiting just to do these first steps. This is especially true if a lot of people arrived around the same time as you. Depending on your health concern and triage level (remember those colours or numbers), you will be asked to wait in a general waiting room, an inside waiting room, or a special examination room. I go into more details about this later in the book. If your health status has changed, or if you decide to leave before seeing a doctor, do tell the Triage Nurse.

Unlike at walk-in clinics or your regular doctor's office, people in the ED are **not** seen in a "first-come, first-served" order. Rather, the ED staff and department think "**worst first.**" The main goal of the ED staff is to check for, rule out, and treat potentially life and limb-threatening conditions **first**. Yes, wait time is one thing we think about when organizing patient flow, but it's not the most important thing. For more on this important topic of waiting, keep reading.

MYTH: "It doesn't look too busy..."

FACT: A front area that isn't packed full of people doesn't mean it will be a quick visit for you!

Often there are inner waiting areas and bottlenecks there.

The ED is predominantly full of people who arrived long before you and who are still waiting to be seen or re-assessed by a doctor.

If you have a low urgency issue, you may get repeatedly "bumped" down the queue by sicker patients—even if they arrive after you. Think strokes, heart attacks, major trauma, active seizures, or severe allergic reactions.

The sickest patients, where any delay in their care could be life-threatening, often arrive to the resuscitation bay through a back entrance. This is usually away from view and earshot of the public entrance and inner waiting areas.

Nurse Assessment

There are usually many more nurses than doctors working in the ED. A nurse tends to be the first person to ask you more detailed questions about why you came to the ED and to confirm your current medications and any allergies. In smaller centres, this nurse may be the same one that you met at triage. In larger centres, this will be a different nurse, sometimes referred to as a "primary nurse" or "most responsible nurse" (MRN) who will be overseeing your care.

The nurse assessment is an important step because:

- They may be able to start some routine tests such as:
  - Blood or urine analysis
  - Electrocardiogram (ECG) (which checks your heart rhythm and can show potential disease)
  - X-rays
- They may be able to offer you some medications for:
  - Pain and fever
  - Nausea and vomiting
  - Itchiness and allergic reactions
  - Extreme anxiety or agitation
- They can move you into the appropriate space, such as a cubicle or stretcher. They can help you change into a hospital gown to make it easier for the doctor to properly examine you.
- They may be able to help keep you comfortable by turning off the light, providing ice chips, or offering a blanket or pillow or splint.
- They may be able to spend more time getting extra information from friends or family who came to the ED with you.
- They may recheck your vital signs.
- They may ask whether your symptoms have changed.
- They can watch for any worsening of your condition while you are waiting.
- They may ask a doctor to see you faster if they feel it's necessary.

- They can take into account special circumstances (for example, needing a translator).

How to Put on a Hospital Gown

I apologize to patients around the world for the hospital gowns we ask you to change into!

They are, admittedly, for the convenience of healthcare providers, and are not designed for dignity, coverage, warmth, fashion, or ease of use. The hospital probably likes these gowns because they fit many different body types and are easy to wash in large volumes. Doctors like them because they allow easier access to the skin surface to listen to your lungs, feel your belly, check for rashes, and see all your extremities. There are times when it's important to check the genital area or to perform a rectal exam, and both are significantly easier when you're wearing a gown.

Unlike a hotel robe, the hospital gown is open in the back, with ties to hold the sides together. Usually, there is one tie for the neck collar area, then another tie just above the waist. Taking off the gown is as easy as untying the two bows and placing it in the nearest dirty linen hamper.

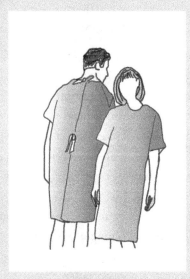

What Do These Numbers and Lines on the Cardiac Monitor Mean?

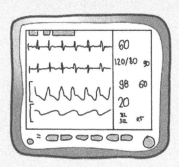

Heart rate – We want to know if your pulse is too slow (under 60 beats/minute) or too fast (over 100 beats/minute), but also if it's irregular or changing to a dangerous rhythm. Stickers on your chest include electrodes that attach to different colored wires connected to the monitor.

Blood pressure – An arm cuff attached to the monitor tightens to check blood pressure periodically. Blood pressure is measured as a higher number and a lower number separated by a line. Low blood pressure is actually more likely to be a problem, as it can be a sign of serious infection, blood loss, or the heart not properly functioning as a pump. High blood pressure tends to be silent and not as worrisome in the short term as most people think. Long-term control of blood pressure helps reduce risks of certain diseases. Your blood pressure goes up and down often and can go up because of pain, stress, worry, or as a side-effect from medications.

Pulse oximetry ("oxygen saturation") – A small clip (a pulse oximeter) is attached to your finger or ear. It shines a red light through your skin and measures the amount of oxygen being carried by your blood. We get concerned when your oxygen saturation drops below 92%. The waveform on the monitor helps us check if the pulse oximeter is picking up the pulse properly, as many things cause a falsely low oxygen saturation reading.

Physician Assessment

As an ED physician, here is how I would approach most of my patients, and you can expect roughly the same from any ED physician. However, I work in a big city ED, where basic and advanced diagnostics, such as CT and ultrasound scans, are available. In smaller or rural centres, and for more specialized tests like MRI or echocardiograms, the ED might not be able to do all the necessary tests at that moment. Staff may have to call patients back to the hospital on another day or at a different location.

First, I would review your patient chart and the results of any tests or imaging ordered by the rest of the team. I would then try to get a focused history of what your main symptoms are, in your own words. I would also ask about certain symptoms to make sure *you didn't* have them and to check for hallmarks of potentially serious illness, even if those diseases are unlikely. You may have answered many of these questions before, but I like to double-check.

Next, I would do a targeted physical examination to look for findings that might rule in or rule out possible causes for the symptoms you have described. "Rule out" is a bit of a simplification; few things can be definitively ruled out. Each piece of information and each test result goes into my overall decision-making process to figure out if a particular diagnosis is more likely or less likely.

If there are specific tests that would help right away, such as a CT scan or blood work, then I would order those. Interestingly, there are some conditions that we simply can't test for. In these cases, I have to figure out if your pattern of signs and symptoms fits into a similar grouping of conditions that we give a certain label, such as "migraine headache" or "irritable bowel syndrome." If I suspected a migraine headache, I might order a CT scan of your brain to make sure it's not a *subarachnoid hemorrhage* ("brain bleed," perhaps from an aneurysm). If I suspected *irritable bowel syndrome*, a CT scan can help me rule out other causes such as *Crohn's colitis* (an autoimmune disease affecting the guts that may need steroid pills to calm down).

Investigations

Once the doctor has at least a partial history of what's ailing you, certain tests may be ordered to help screen for possible causes. Frequently performed tests include blood work, imaging tests, an ECG, or a urinalysis. Each of these involves multiple steps to request, perform, and process, so it takes time to get the results to your ED doctor. Sometimes, behind the scenes, other doctors are helping to figure out what is normal versus abnormal. A pathologist might have to examine your blood more carefully under a microscope. A radiologist will be doing a formal report on your X-ray or CT scan based on what they see, previous imaging tests, and the reason for the new exam.

The common theme of a number of tests performed in the ED is based on the question "will the result change the management of your care?" If not, then that testing doesn't need to be done—or at least not right away. Perhaps the treatment would be the same no matter what the test result might show.

It's important to note that some routine tests that your Family Doctor might order are *not* best done during your ED visit. Particular tests need to happen under certain circumstances, such as on an empty stomach, with a full bladder, or timed around medications.

Common Investigations Explained

In the ED, we utilize several tests to help us see what is going on below the surface. We can then see bones, muscles, organs, and more. These tests can help us detect health problems and make more accurate diagnoses.

- **CT Scan** (computed tomography scan)

A CT machine spins an X-ray generator and sensors to provide a 3D view of internal organs and structures. The patient is placed on a sliding platform that briefly moves through a round doughnut-shaped portal. The images obtained are quite detailed and help us tell, for example, if there has been a recent stroke or bleeding in the brain, a blood clot in the lungs, or infections in the abdomen such as appendicitis or diverticulitis.

- **ECG/EKG** (electrocardiogram)

This quick, simple, cheap, and non-invasive test gives us a snapshot of your heart and how it is beating. Stickers are applied to your chest and limbs and the electrical signals are recorded and printed out. It can demonstrate if you are having (or have ever had) a heart attack. But it can also give us clues about your electrolytes, show arrhythmias, warn us to *not* use certain medications, or hint at other life-threatening conditions.

- **MRI** (magnetic resonance imaging)

Finer detail can in many instances be achieved with an MRI, and different from what a CT scan can show. Some things, such as bone and blood, may be seen less well than on CT. The benefit of this test is that no radiation is used. However, it can be slower, less accessible, and louder than other tests. The tube of an MRI machine where a patient goes into is a longer tunnel, so claustrophobia is more of an issue for an MRI compared to a CT scan.

- **Ultrasound**

This imaging test uses sound waves, like sonar in a submarine, instead of X-rays to look deep inside the body. In certain cases in the ED, we use "bedside ultrasound" for a quick look inside, like a visual stethoscope. There is also a comprehensive version we call a "formal ultrasound," which is done by a technician and read by a radiologist, but they tend to be booked during standard business hours. Ultrasounds are safe for every patient because there is no radiation involved, so we prefer to use them in kids when we are worried about appendicitis, for example, or for testing in pregnant women.

- **X-Ray**

Using low doses of radiation, X-rays can give us a snapshot of certain parts of the body very quickly. The waves pass through differently depending on whether there is bone or air or fluid in the way before reaching a detector. We can easily see if a bone is broken, a lung is collapsed, or if there is fluid where there normally shouldn't be. Sometimes we get enough clues to help us figure out what is going on, such as X-ray patterns suggesting a bowel blockage or rupture. We used to have to look at actual X-ray "films" that were like giant black and white photos; but just as photography has become digital, now we can see the processed X-ray images on a computer screen.

Treatment

In Canada, there are over 15 million ED visits a year.[1] The true number is actually much higher because several regions provide incomplete data or none at all. In the USA, there are over 138 million visits annually—a shocking 43 visits for every 100 persons![2]

Although we do perform resuscitations for people coming in when their hearts stop beating properly (*cardiac arrest*) or they can't get enough air to breathe (*respiratory arrest*), most of the day-to-day treatments we provide in the ED are for pain, nausea, worry, and injury. We try to stabilize a patient's acute medical problems and move them along a treatment journey when it is safer to do so. ED doctors provide "episodic care" meaning we do not routinely do "continuing care" or follow-up outside of our six- to twelve-hour shift.

The top five problems leading to ED visits in Canada, in order, are

1) Abdominal and pelvic pain

---

1   Canadian Institute for Health Information. *NACRS Emergency Department Visits and Length of Stay by Province/Territory, 2018–2019*. Ottawa, ON: CIHI, 2019. Table 1.

2   Rui P., Kang K. *National Hospital Ambulatory Medical Care Survey: 2017 emergency department summary tables*. National Center for Health Statistics. https://www.cdc.gov/nchs/data/nhamcs/web_tables/2017_ed_web_tables-508.pdf.

2) Chest and throat pain
3) Respiratory tract infections
4) Back pain
5) Urinary tract disease

Wounds, skin infections, and gastrointestinal disease are also in the top 10.[3] I discuss all of these problems at some point in this book.

Here are some examples of treatments we perform for common conditions.

Condition	Treatment	Method
Anaphylaxis (severe allergy)	Calm the immune response	Epinephrine plus antihistamine and steroid medications. May be given into the muscles, veins, mouth, or lungs, depending on the situation
Anemia	Blood transfusion	Given slowly through an intravenous (IV) line
Asthma / COPD attack	Improve breathing and oxygen levels	Inhaled medications to open up the lungs, steroids to calm the inflammation and spasm, extra oxygen or breathing support
Bleeding nose that won't stop (epistaxis)	Internal pressure, sometimes cauterization	Topical freezing, inserting a balloon device or tightly packed gauze. Chemical or electrical "burning" (cauterization) of a blood vessel if we can spot it.

---

3   Canadian Institute for Health Information. *NACRS Emergency Department Visits and Length of Stay by Province/Territory, 2018–2019*. Ottawa, ON: CIHI, 2019. Table 6a.

Broken bone (*fracture*)	Straighten and immobilize the injury	After some sedation*, pulling the bone back into position, applying a plaster or fibreglass cast or splint (a partial cast)
Cut (*laceration*)	Close the wound	Stitches (deep dissolvable and/or skin-level removable). Medical tape, staples, or glue
Diabetic complications: e.g. coma, confusion, acidic blood	Normalize blood sugar	IV dextrose if blood sugar is too low. Insulin if blood sugar is too high
Dehydration (severe)	Rehydrate	Sometimes IV electrolytes and medications until pills and sips of fluids stay down
Dislocation	Putting the bone back into joint	After some sedation*, manipulation of the bone
Heart attack	Restore blood flow to an acutely blocked blood vessel	"Clot-busting" IV medications and/or rapid transfer to a cardiologist for balloon and stent procedure
Hypothermia	Rewarm	Warmed fluids, a heated forced-air blanket
Migraine and other headaches	Reduce pain and nausea	Multiple medications, often IV if the patient can't keep pills or sips down
Overdose (for example, heroin/opioid)	Restore ability to breathe	Naloxone antidote
Poisoning	Supportive care or active treatment	Antidote, if available
Seizures	Stop the seizure if it doesn't stop on its own	Antiseizure medication injection
Sepsis (severe infection)	Combat the overwhelming infection	IV fluids, antibiotics, finding and controlling the source

Stroke	Restore blood flow to the brain if recent enough	"Clot-busting" IV medications and/or rapid transfer for clot-retrieval with new technology
Urinary obstruction	Drain the bladder	Insert a catheter attached to a urine collection bag

* For some necessary procedures, the doctor will offer medication so the patient doesn't feel or remember the event. Depending on the doctor's experience and the setting, they may be able to use an IV medication that only takes minutes to work, and wears off very quickly.

Scared of Needles?

Everyone has their kryptonite. Mine is bugs. Blood and guts and bodily fluids don't chase me away, but a creepy-crawly that could get near my neck? Count me out!

If your kryptonite is the thought or sight of getting poked with a needle, here a few tricks to help:

- **Cough** – Ask the doctor or nurse to insert the needle at the same time that you cough. For example, on the count of three, "1, 2, 3, cough!"

- **Pinch** – As the needle is about to go in, use your other hand to pinch yourself firmly somewhere else, such as on your thigh or waist. Focus on the pain you are creating and can control. Pinch harder if you need to.

- **Breathe** – Before the needle goes in, take deep breaths in and blow away the pain loudly through pursed lips. This helps because we tend to breathe shallowly and tightly when stressed.

Discharge

Emergency doctors often think of the last step first. What I mean is that from the minute we sign up for a patient, we ask ourselves what their "disposition" is likely to be. Is this someone who needs to be admitted to the hospital for acute treatment and more investigation or is this someone who can go home today?

We treat many patients and often send them home. These include patients with a cut we can repair, an asthma attack that we can stabilize and treat with home medications, or a broken bone that we can X-ray and put in a cast.

Examples of patients who need to be admitted include someone with appendicitis that requires surgery, someone who is frail and falling for some reason and isn't safe to be at home, or someone with pneumonia that is so severe that they need oxygen.

Most people can be discharged from the ED—approximately 80% of arrivals in my standard workweek. That's not to say that we diagnose or fix a high percentage of people who come through the doors. Unfortunately, many people leave *without* a clear-cut diagnosis even after all our tests. Patients undoubtedly feel frustrated when we can't explain their symptoms and they feel no further ahead after spending so long in the ED.

As a rule, we can move people one or two steps forward on their path of figuring out what might be causing their symptoms and how to treat them. But we tend to see only a snapshot, and that may not be enough to piece together the whole puzzle. Perhaps the answers will become more obvious with time. Or maybe trial and error with different medications is necessary. It might be helpful to see a specialist; however, they may not be readily available for everyone who comes through the ED, and it can sometimes take a while to see them in their office.

Having a family doctor or nurse practitioner in your community who can see you over time is extremely valuable. They have the benefit of knowing your health story, your family, your preferences, your personal circumstances, and personality. They can see all the different pieces of your personal health jigsaw puzzle and put them together, see what fits and what doesn't, and explain it to you along the way.

What If You Don't Have a Family Doctor?

Unfortunately, in many parts of Canada, it is getting more difficult to find a community doctor, for reasons that are beyond what I can cover in this book. If you have one, consider yourself lucky and thank them for being there for you! If not, do try to use the same walk-in or urgent care clinic so your records are all in one place. You may see a different face each time you go, but at least the reasons you sought medical care, as well as the findings and treatment plans, will be accessible to the doctor.

There are new telehealth or virtual clinics available, but keep in mind the doctors there will likely be unable to examine you or do a complete assessment. They can order lab work, X-rays, prescribe or refill medications, counsel you for mental health issues, and also help you determine if you need to go to the ED.

Admission

Where I practice, approximately one in five people who come to the ED require admission to the hospital for further investigations, treatment, surgery, or palliative care.

After your physician assessment and investigations are done, the doctor may decide that it's not safe for you to go home. Typically, the next step would be to admit you to the hospital under the care of a specific physician or "most responsible physician" (MRP).

In an ideal world, you would quickly be transferred to your designated "inpatient bed" in a different part of the hospital. Sadly, in many facilities around the world, the hospital may be full or even over-capacity. That is, there are more people needing a hospital bed than there are physical spaces and staff to care for them.

The result is that some people get stuck in the ED or a hallway waiting for a bed "upstairs" to free up. In Canada, the average time ED patients spend waiting for an inpatient bed has gone up over the years and sits at over 24 hours. Sadly, I've even witnessed loved ones of mine unable to get a bed, admitted to hospital but staying on an emergency stretcher, for several days!

"Board to Tears"

The practice of keeping patients in the ED who belong elsewhere in the hospital is sometimes called "boarding" and it is a real problem from coast to coast. It impacts new patient arrivals to the ED who get stuck in our hallways if it's the only spot to place them. We can't do a proper examination or have private discussions there.

Emergency nurses are occupied doing tasks and giving medications to admitted patients who could be looked after elsewhere in the hospital, instead of bringing in new patients from the waiting room and assessing them.

What Is the Emergency Department NOT Good At?

Much of the time there are more people seeking service through the ED than there is space or providers to care for them in an ideal way. We have no control over how many people arrive and when, how sick they are, and how many need to be admitted. Our healthcare colleagues habitually say to their patients, "If things get worse, go to Emerg." And while we are proud to be the safety net for the community, it's impossible to be everything for everyone at all hours. Even when I start my shift with the best of intentions, I regularly end up wishing some things could have been handled differently. Chiefly our departments are designed for function, so other factors are not prioritized, or the ED may not be the ideal place or have the best clinicians to handle certain issues.

- **Privacy**: Don't be surprised if you are able to hear snippets of someone else's medical issues. Your personal and sensitive information may be overheard by others. We try to limit how often this happens and try to be discreet about as much as we can. Please respect other patients' privacy by not repeating anything you have seen or heard about another patient.
- **Quiet**: People of all ages are sometimes loud when they are upset, in pain, intoxicated, or in distress. Nurses might have to yell into a deaf patient's ear to be heard. Alerts and alarms are going off all the time. Doctors might be talking loudly into their phones or dictation machines. Staff quickly get used to the cacophony of groans, crying children, beeps, dings, and simultaneous conversations. I feel sorry for the patient coming in for a migraine headache with photophonophobia (bothered by sound and light)!
- **Dignity**: Patient gowns don't offer much coverage, warmth, or fashion. Washrooms are shared. Bedside commodes aren't always emptied fast enough. The ED may be unable to accommodate all family members wanting to be beside a dying loved one. A thin

curtain may be the only thing separating a person at the end of their life from a foul-smelling or a loud psychotic individual.

- **Chronic conditions**: If it's been going on for a long time, we in the ED may not be the best providers to help since we're giving "episodic care." Whether it's mental health, a social situation, chronic pain, or a problematic joint, we may not know what has already been tried. It can be tricky trying to step into the middle of a diagnostic/therapeutic process that another doctor may have started. I try to provide temporary symptom relief, perhaps some more information or resources, and at least help move people a step further on their path. But I may not be able to give you the time, attention, or follow-up that you need. We try to address the "chief complaint" and issues that may be tied into it; however, we cannot take a fully comprehensive approach to multiple concerns when there is a long lineup of people waiting to be seen and attended to. If you have a GP, they are a specialist in Family Medicine and you benefit from the continuity of someone being able to care for you over the long term.

- **Infections**: We try to isolate people with diseases that we know are airborne or transmitted by droplets and direct touch. However, a lot of sick people come through our doors including possible cases of tuberculosis, measles, Norwalk virus, chickenpox, influenza, or a host of other infectious diseases. Thanks to dedicated housekeeping staff, patient care areas are cleaned regularly. Still, if you didn't have something *before* you came to the hospital, there is a chance you might leave with an unwanted souvenir you pick up there. Whether you're a patient or a support person, you can help yourself and everyone around you by washing your hands frequently (or by using sanitizer) before, during, and after your visit. If you have a cough, wear a mask to limit the spread of droplets to those around you.

- **Moving you from the ED into the rest of the hospital:** If you are unfortunate enough to be so ill that you require admission to hospital by the emergency physician, you may spend over 24 hours in the ED waiting to be transferred to a room or bed in the part of the hospital called "units," "floors," or "wards."

- **Fixing other parts of the health care system:** We ordinarily cannot get you a Family Doctor if you've been unable to find one that accepts patients in your community. We cannot speed things up if you are on a waiting list to see a specialist, get an MRI, or have a surgical procedure. Exceptions are based on the medical situation, not a special power we have compared to the doctors outside the hospital.

Why See a Family Doctor?

Evidence shows that long-term care from a family doctor leads to fewer hospitalizations, lower mortality, better overall health outcomes, and higher satisfaction with your health care.

Family doctors specialize in providing whole-person, patient-centred care that improves your quality of life and addresses any physical or mental health concerns. An ongoing relationship with your family doctor means there is someone who knows you well and can help you stay healthy through all stages of your life.

Find out more at https://bccfp.bc.ca/myfamilydoctorcares/

What are Emergency Personnel Not Good At?

- **Provider self-care:** Staff go into healthcare professions to help people, and when there are so many ill and suffering patients, staff often skip breaks, delay bathroom breaks until bursting, and try to catch up on paperwork while they shovel what they can into their mouths. We should know better than to perpetuate these unhealthy habits. The irony is that sometimes healthcare workers don't take care of themselves—to the point where they become less effective, less patient, or seem less caring. Earlier in my career, I tried to work as fast as possible. It was disheartening to start my shift with a three-hour department wait time, work as hard as I could, and then leave with a four-hour wait time for patients to see a doctor! For me, rebalancing meant slowing down a bit to spend that extra minute with a patient and family, to offer a warm greeting to the team around me, and to stay fed and hydrated on-shift. Instead of aiming to see as many patients as I could, I changed my perspective to one of leaving the world a slightly better place than when I arrived that day.

PART 2
HURRY UP... AND WAIT

Why Are You Waiting So Long?

Across the nation, the average time from when you arrive at the ED to when you will see a doctor is over three hours.[4] There are many factors that affect how long an individual patient will have to wait. As a result, it's difficult and often inaccurate to estimate that "it will be a four-hour wait," for example. Even though *you* may prefer to know the possible wait time before you register, trying to predict that for every person may occasionally scare away someone who really needs to stay! For example, we see people presenting in the middle of having a heart attack. Now and then, they don't realize how serious their symptoms actually are—or we only recognize it after initial testing like an ECG. If they had thought it was certain to take a very long time to see a doctor, they may have returned home too soon. Sometimes I joke with patients that *it's a good thing* they weren't rushed in! From our perspective, those folks who are brought straight in to see a doctor are the ones at risk of dying before being able to leave the ED.

Even if you are the next person by "length of stay" (LOS) to be seen, you might get "bumped" by a trauma ("blunt" like a motor vehicle collision or "penetrating" like a stabbing). Often a patient with a serious heart attack or potential stroke may arrive and need to be assessed as soon as possible.

Critical patients in the trauma bay also require more team members at the bedside, so staff are necessarily pulled away from other parts of the ED to help out. One very sick patient can tie up almost all the department's resources.

---

4   Canadian Institute for Health Information. *NACRS Emergency Department Visits and Length of Stay by Province/Territory, 2018–2019*. Ottawa, ON: CIHI, 2019. Table 9.

Visits by Triage Scale

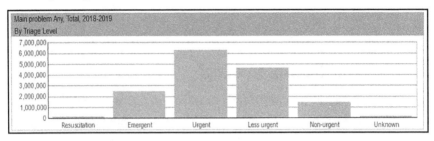

Main problem Any, Total, 2018-2019
By Triage Level

This table shows that the majority of the people who come to get checked out are in the medium-risk category when assessed by the Triage Nurse.[5] Those in the categories in the middle and on the right tend to get bumped by patients arriving with a triage category of "resuscitation" and "emergent" on the left.

Perhaps the doctor isn't occupied with diagnosing a life, limb, or vision-threatening condition. Perhaps they are delivering bad news such as discovering a tumour that might be cancer or asking a family whether their loved one has any wishes about end-of-life care. It's best not to rush important conversations like these. Some patient conversations take longer. As another example, we sometimes have to communicate via a translator, which can take twice as long.

Yes, it's frustrating to wait. And perhaps it is disappointing to not be able to spend a long time talking to the doctor when it is your turn. Your doctor wants to serve you with high-quality care, and yet they are also worried about a potential "ticking time-bomb" type of condition in patients sitting in the waiting room that no one has seen yet. So, we have to balance those competing needs.

---

5   Canadian Institute for Health Information. *NACRS Emergency Department (ED) Visits: Volumes and Median Length of Stay by Triage Level, Visit Disposition, and Main Problem, 2018–2019*. Accessed July 31, 2020. https://www.cihi.ca/en/nacrs-emergency-depart-ment-ed-visits-volumes-and-median-length-of-stay-by-triage-level-visit.

Please Do Not Keep Asking the Nurses How Long It Will Be!

It can be hard to estimate how long your individual wait will be.

When several people in the waiting areas ask this question, it takes time away from other duties the nurse has including:

- Filling orders the physician has requested
- Getting patients ready to be seen in an appropriate setting
- Discharging patients who are ready to go home
- Communicating in writing or verbally with other team members
- Being pulled into the trauma room or
- Covering for another nurse who is occupied.

Sometimes patients leave moments before the doctor is able to see them, perhaps fed up with the wait or perhaps being told it was going to be another hour or two of waiting.

Why Did That Other Person Get Called Before You?

In addition to the factors above, there are several other reasons why patients may be called out of order from a strict "length of stay" perspective.

Test Results Can Take Time

Certain test results, such as lab work and X-rays, take a while to come back. A nurse may have initiated those and the doctor can better serve you by waiting until those initial results are available.

Returning and "Pre-Arrival" Patients

Sometimes we ask patients to return the next day for more tests or treatments. Since these patients waited just as long the day before, and because they have a plan in place already, we might see them more quickly. Similarly, if a physician refers you to the ED and speaks with an emergency doctor over the phone, you can be entered as a "pre-arrival" in our computers. Although not guaranteed, we may see you sooner since we already know a bit of the story and action plan.

Waiting for the Most Appropriate Examination Room

The most appropriate room for your condition may not be available yet. For example, eye rooms have specialized equipment and medications, procedure rooms may offer better lighting and more space to work, and gynecological rooms have special stretchers to allow for pelvic exams and swabs if necessary. Perhaps the room you need is being cleaned, but a simple room is available for someone with a different presenting illness or injury. (For more about different rooms in the ED, please see page **54, "Basic Emergency Department Layout"**).

Doctor Decisions

Doctor-related factors and preferences can also affect whom they choose to see next. For example, if I'm aware of a patient from a previous visit, or a conversation with a colleague, it might be more straightforward for me to see that person instead of another doctor who doesn't have that knowledge.

A doctor might be waiting for results on multiple sick patients. He or she may not be able to start another complex case, but perhaps can see a minor case that doesn't need as much time or brainpower, or that can be easily put on hold. Taking this one patient out of order means everyone gets seen a little bit faster.

Shift Changes

Where I work, there can be four or more emergency physicians working at the same time, with overlapping shifts. Whoever is at the end of their shift mainly sees the more straightforward-sounding cases. So, you might notice the doctor who is about to finish their shift start seeing cases like sprains and cuts out of order, ahead of chest pain or abdominal pain patients. This is good for everybody, because at the end of a long shift when I'm tired, hungry, and looking at the clock, I'm not as sharp. That's how errors happen. Mistakes can also happen when cases are "handed over" to the incoming physician. So, if you might need advanced imaging tests (that may take hours longer to get and be reported on), it may be better for you to be seen by a fresh physician who has enough time left in their shift to see you through to completion.

ED Physicians Are Also Teachers

Learners regularly rotate through the ED and work with staff physicians. In addition to medical students and residents, there may be nursing and para-medic students. They are all getting practical "on the job" training and may be directed to certain case presentations by their supervisor. Each learner will have unique capabilities and learning needs. So, a junior medical student, full of book knowledge but a novice in the real world, may not be able to see highly complex patients, but rather the more "bread and butter" or "classic textbook" presentations.

A more senior learner rotating through the ED, such as a military medic or a rural GP coming in for additional training, may be trying to focus on a particular type of case. For example, if they are trying to expand their orthopedic knowledge, they might try to see all the cases involving broken bones, dislocated joints, sprains, and lacerations—regardless of how long that patient has been waiting.

Patients or Patience?

It is difficult and stressful to wait, especially when you are suffering or in pain, but please be polite and respectful with the staff.

We are all doing our best to care for everyone in a timely manner.

Your cooperation helps us do our job to the best of our ability.

If you are on an emergency stretcher, consider using the "emergency call bell" for urgent issues such as pain, nausea, dizziness, or breathing problems. For comfort and convenience questions (such as requests for a warm blanket, a drink of water, a box of tissues, adjustments of the pillow, or changing the angle of the bed) please save these for when your nurse comes to the bedside. Your emergency nurse will frequently check with you when they are not busy with another patient.

How to Speed Up Your Visit and Streamline Your Care

These tips aren't guaranteed to reduce your length of stay, but from my experience, can certainly make a difference. Some of these suggestions may surprise you.

Figure Out How to Describe Your Symptoms

Much of the information we need to make a diagnosis is based on the history of your presenting illness. Try to find a way to summarize why you are seeking emergency medical care in ten words or less. If the triage nurse asks you, "what brings you here?" you should have a quick answer ready that isn't "Because my doctor sent me!"

You will be asked for more detail later during your ED visit.

If you have pain, check out page **69** for details your emergency doctor will want to know. Giving this *OPQRST* can reduce the number of questions you are asked.

Ask Before You Pee!

Urine tests are sometimes very helpful, and if the doctor is waiting for a sample to be collected and analyzed, it can sometimes prolong your visit by hours! If you are a female of childbearing age, we will want to make sure you are not pregnant before doing certain tests or giving certain medications. In other cases, doctors might need to do an ultrasound and want you to have a relatively full bladder to get a better quality scan.

Urine samples are *especially* useful if you have any of the following symptoms:

- Urinary issues such as pain or having to pee frequently.
- Discharge (unusual fluid) coming from your penis or vagina.
- Fever or nausea without a clear cause.
- Back pain or trauma. Kidney problems often cause pain to be felt in your back

- Abdominal (stomach area) or pelvic pain or trauma.
- Unusual rashes or fever. Sometimes the urine sample can show microscopic blood or protein that can give us clues about the cause.

How to Collect a Good Urine Sample

Urine that touches the skin before reaching the container can be contaminated and cause false readings. We ask patients to get a good "clean catch" from mid-stream urine.

The basic steps are:

- Ask the nurse if a urine specimen is needed so they can give you a container.

- Prepare the container in the washroom by removing the lid and placing it somewhere protected from getting splashed.

- Clean the genital skin, starting with the urethra (where the urine comes out).

- Because the first bit of urine to come out is the dirtiest, start urinating as you normally would, and **try to catch the middle of the stream—** neither the beginning nor the end.

- Screw the lid on **tightly**, since leaking containers may not be processed by the lab

- You may be asked to put a **label** or write your **name** on it, so your nurse knows it is yours.

- There may be a designated location to place a collected specimen. Otherwise, return it to a nurse when they are available.

Like at many offices and clinics, some urine analysis can be done with a quick **dipstick**, which only takes a few minutes. Other times, a laboratory technician must analyze the urine under a **microscope**, which takes longer.

A crucial test is the **urine culture**, for which a sample is plated on a petri dish to see if any bacteria grow. This process can take days to provide the information needed. These cultures help doctors discover what **bug** is there, what **drug** will work against it (sensitivity), and what the bug is **resistant** to (resistances).

Ask Before You Eat or Drink Much!

Sips of water are probably OK, but some tests are best done on an empty stomach, and some procedures are safer that way too. Some conditions, such as pancreatitis or a bowel obstruction, could be made worse by adding any food to your digestive system.

Have Your Medical History and List of Medications Written Down

We will ask you repeatedly about previous illnesses, surgeries, pregnancies, and medications. It's very useful if this information is written down. Some patients find it helpful to bring their medications in their original pill bottles or blister packs. Unlabelled pills are rarely beneficial for us to see because there are dozens of look-alikes.

See Appendix 3 for a sample medical history summary that you can fill in and keep with you whenever you need to go to the ED.

Provide Names and Contact Information for Your Other Medical Specialists

If you have seen any medical specialists in the last year, it can be helpful to provide their names. This is especially true if you want us to try to send them any information from your visit.

Do Tell!

Your primary nurse is often the team member who is most familiar with your case, so please let them know about any of the following:

- **Any new symptoms** that weren't there when you first came in, such as fever, severe pain or nausea, rash or itch, or feeling like you are about to faint.

- **If you are leaving.** Whether you are stepping out to pay for parking or choosing to seek care elsewhere, please let us know. When the staff have to spend time calling out names, or trying to locate people who have left, they are using valuable time that could be spent caring for other patients.

What If You Are Not Sure About Whether You Should Go to the ED?

To be safe, if you are worried, come in any time. But if you are not sure, here are a few options to try first:

Check in With Your FP/GP

If you have an FP/GP, they may have appointments reserved for patients who need to be seen that same day. If you are sick outside of office hours (evenings, nights, weekends, holidays) their clinic may have an after-hours physician on-call who will speak to you.

Consider Other Options Like Your Local Pharmacist

For less urgent issues, they can suggest over-the-counter medications and check for drug interactions with your existing prescriptions. A surprising number of people go to the ED for issues such as constipation, itch, hemorrhoids, vaginal yeast infections, pinworms, or lice that could have been managed by a pharmacist. They might also offer clinics for managing blood pressure, diabetes, vaccinations, and smoking cessation.

Call Your Province's Healthcare Info Line

In some provinces, there are free services that provide advice over the phone. You can speak to a nurse about your symptoms and get advice on the best way to proceed.

- British Columbia, Alberta, Saskatchewan, Quebec, New Brunswick, Nova Scotia, Prince Edward Island, and Newfoundland and Labrador: Call 8-1-1
- Manitoba: Call 1-888-315-9257
- Ontario: Call 1-866-797-0000

Of course, it can be difficult for a nurse or physician to make a definitive decision over the phone. To be safe, they may advise you to go to the ED.

You could reply with the question, "when?" Do they think you need to go immediately, or could you possibly wait until the morning? They might tell you, "if it gets worse, or doesn't get any better, then go to the emergency."

There's more to 8-1-1 Than a Nurse!

In addition to tele-health advice and answering questions about how to navigate the health system in your area, some regions provide additional services through 811, such as:

- Registered dietitian

- Pharmacist

- Exercise professionals

- Dementia advice

- Osteoporosis screening

- Addictions information and referrals

- Health information topics available online

- Ability to discuss health information in dozens of languages, depending on the availability of translators.

Search the Internet for more information about the 811 program in your province.

In an interview for a CBC article, Halifax healthcare consultant Mary Jane Hampton had the following to say about 8-1-1 Health Link services in Nova Scotia:

> Hampton said the 811 service is panned by those who assume that due to liability issues, the nurses on the line will probably just advise you to go to the emergency department, whatever the issue.
>
> "That's actually not true," she said. "About 19 percent of calls do end up with the 811 nurse saying, 'It does sound to me like you should go to the emergency department, so head on over.'
>
> "But, the really interesting statistics are that about 42 percent of people who call in are told that the reason that they phoned is

certainly something that warrants making an appointment to see your family doctor or a nurse practitioner, but it's not an emergency.

"Here's the really neat statistic: About 30 percent of calls end up with the 811 nurse being able to give advice and information to the person about how to manage the condition themselves.

"When you consider that 42 percent of people are potentially being saved an unnecessary visit to an emergency department or walk-in clinic, and almost a third of people are being told that they don't need to go anywhere else, they can safely manage the issue—that's what makes the 811 service really powerful, and that's where it becomes a really important tool in helping to navigate the system."[6]

---

6   "How to make the most of 811," CBC News, May 7, 2019, https://www.cbc.ca/news/canada/nova-scotia/how-to-make-the-most-of-the-811-service-1.5126002.

Is There a Good Time of Day to Visit So You Wait Less?

It's rare that the urban ED is "quiet." In fact, there is strong superstition about this word. If we utter the "Q word" we often get a disapproving stare or a loudly whispered "Shhh!" from the staff.

Weekdays, on the whole, start out less busy. Quickly though, community doctors start referring patients they are worried about. Workers start injuring themselves on the job or during their commutes. Our ED gets progressively fuller and wait times go up. By the time regular doctors' offices close, there are fewer options for the unwell, and we consistently see the number of people registering continue to go up through the day. Coughs seem to get worse in the evening and children seem to get fussier then too, so parents predictably arrive at that time wanting a doctor to check their little ones out. It can take until the night shift to finish assessing and treating the backlog of patients. Commonly, it's not until the wee hours of the night before we feel "caught up" from the day. Then the cycle repeats!

Fridays, weekends, and holidays can be extra busy. There may not be anywhere else to turn except the ED. In the midst of these peak times, it can be disheartening for staff to see a patient who has had their problem for months, and who chooses to come on a Monday of a long weekend for their convenience, when that person could have just made an appointment to see a doctor in the community.

Why Can't You Lie Down Somewhere? Can You Stay in a Stretcher?

Unfortunately, there are many more people who arrive each day than there are stretchers to see them in. At the hospitals I work in, we might see 200 people a day. Stretchers are generally reserved for people who need continuous heart monitoring, isolation because they might have an infectious disease, specialized tests, sedation for a procedure, or those who are too ill to stand. In order to assess and treat people as efficiently as possible, we do a bit of "musical chairs." People who can walk or have someone who can help them in the "ambulatory" care area might move into one room for the first assessment, then move to another area for lab work or an ECG, and somewhere else for treatments. Between these steps, they may spend their time waiting in an inner waiting area.

Sadly, hospitals are often over-capacity, and it can be difficult to move patients who need to be admitted into a bed in one of the hospital wards. That backup or "bed block" gets felt in the overcrowded ED as those patients stay stuck on stretchers, slowing our ability to see new patients, and occupying ED staff. Meanwhile, the lineup in the waiting room grows.

If You're Getting Really Anxious and Distressed While Waiting, What Can You Do?

Here are three things you can do in the ED, but also at home, work, school when you're getting more emotionally distressed:

1. **Ice pack trick** – Close your eyes while you place something as cold as you can stand (like a frozen gel pack) for as long as you can stand it right over your eyeballs and forehead. We use this trick in little kids with abnormally fast heart rates. It's amazing—this works so quickly that we can see the heart rate come down on the heart monitor. We think it works by triggering the "diving reflex." Basically, if you fell through the ice on a frozen lake and plunged into the water, your body would go into "mini-hibernation." Your body instinctively slows everything down to protect your vital organs. I call it "anti-adrenaline."

   Combine this method with holding your breath for short periods, or try pairing it with one of the methods below.

2. **Progressive muscle tensing and de-tensing** – First, try tensing up muscles as tightly as you can. These muscles could be the ones in your hands, arms, legs, feet, or even face. Try tensing them up so hard that your limbs start to tremble, and hold for five seconds. Then let your entire body relax and go limp for at least five seconds. Repeat this as many times as you want, seeing if you can involve even more muscles than the time before.

3. **Relaxation breaths** – My kids learned these in school as "square breathing" because each of these four steps should take about the same length of time—about four seconds. If you want something easy to remember:

   - Take a slow deep breath IN counting silently to yourself "IN-two-three-four."

   - Next, HOLD your full breath saying in your head "HOLD-two-three-four."

   - Then, slowly breathe OUT over four seconds, counting "OUT-two-three-four."

   - Finally, HOLD your empty breath quietly thinking "HOLD-two-three-four."

Repeat this cycle over and over with your eyes closed.

Why Do You Have to Tell Your Story Again and Again?

While you're at the ED, you may feel like you're being asked the same questions over and over. You are. But it's important for several reasons:

Different objectives. Each team member may have a different priority, whether that is to sort out who needs immediate attention, to treat any symptoms while the wait continues, to diagnose your condition, to reassess your illness, to properly identify you for the tests being requested, or to assess your safety and ability to return home.

So we don't miss important details! Often a nurse might catch something that I didn't, or a patient may remember a new part of their story that they forgot to mention earlier. Some information, such as allergies, is so important that we like to double (and triple) check.

Better understanding. Ultimately, your health and what matters to you is clearer when your healthcare provider hears it directly from you. Second-hand information may be OK in a summary, but just like in the "broken telephone game," errors can occur when information is passed on from one person to another. In fact, if things really aren't making sense to me, I might have to go back and ask questions I didn't ask the first time. Perhaps I ask them in a different way or ask family members to clarify.

Hospitals are teaching environments. "Doctor" is a word derived from the Latin "to teach," and I would not be able to do my job if it hadn't been for experienced physicians supervising me in clinics and in hospitals across the country. Now I have the privilege of trying to pass on some of my knowledge and advice to the next generation of doctors. As a patient, you might see any (or all three) of the medical student, resident, or staff physician, and all of them will need to ask you questions.

PART 3
PEOPLE AND PLACES

Why I Love Being an Emergency Physician

One of the reasons I love my job is the variety of patients and issues that I see every shift. Although it is humbling to regularly see things I have never seen before, or to prepare for worst-case situations that may never happen, the challenge of this work is important and enriching. It brings me meaning *because* it is difficult.

I Never Know What I'm Going to See When I Start My Day

At any time, someone might arrive with a serious illness, injuries and broken bones, a mental health crisis, an exotic infection, or a rare genetic disorder. We see people from all walks and stages of life—newborns, the elderly, travellers from afar, the homeless, pregnant women, and even staff from other departments in the hospital.

I Work with a Variety of Dedicated Team Members

I am so grateful to all the hardworking people doing their best to help patients. Behind the scenes, they are making sure the department flows, safeguarding against errors I might make, and helping people get home safely. They work long hours and often have to sacrifice a regular meal break or even getting to the bathroom! I might not say "thank you" enough, but I hope my appreciation and respect come through.

The ED team is also the point of contact for ambulance crews and police officers who bring folks to the hospital. We interact with almost every other specialist physician in our region and get to know their quirks and expertise.

I Must Be Adept at Multiple Skills

I must be ready to set a bone, defibrillate a heart, drain a fluid-filled chest, calm a child, counsel a grieving family, or stitch up a wound. I have to be skilled at computers, pattern recognition, and communication—working quickly, yet with kindness and respect.

Who Are All These People?

I am very grateful to work in a team environment where everybody has a vital role to play. But for patients, it can be confusing to figure out who does what. In an ideal world, everyone would be wearing a distinct uniform, with an ID name tag, and introduce themselves to you. In reality, many of us wear scrubs (also known as "greens" since they are traditionally this colour) because they are clean and comfortable! Confusingly, we all then blend together because we're wearing the same color. If you're wondering what someone's role in the ED is, don't ever hesitate to ask them.

Here's a short description of the different people who help me do my job, catch my errors, and care for your health in an urban ED:

- **Nurses**

    - **Triage nurse:** Generally, the first person you see. They will gather a small amount of key information and check your vital signs (such as your temperature, pulse rate, and blood pressure) to determine how serious your condition is or may potentially be.
    - **Charge nurse:** Has a sense of the whole unit, staff, incoming and outgoing flow of patients, resources and shortages, roadblocks, and personalities. Different than your primary nurse.
    - **Primary nurse:** In some EDs, there are too many patients for one nurse to handle. In these EDs, the workload is divided so that one nurse is more familiar with certain patients or certain areas of the department. As a patient, this nurse should be your main point of contact. You are their main responsibility.
    - **Liaison nurse:** Larger centres may have a nurse who collaborates with home and community care nurses. This is helpful for elderly patients who are having difficulty looking after themselves or their partner.

- **Paramedics**

    - There is sometimes a line-up of patients on stretchers waiting with the ambulance attendants who brought them in. In some regions, after patients are triaged, paramedics are allowed to hand over responsibility for patients to the ED. In other regions, ambulance personnel must stay with the patient until that patient ends up in an appropriate emergency bed.

    - Some patients are not able to get home on their own or in a taxi. These patients sometimes need an ambulance equivalent to take them home.

- **Clerks**

    - **Registration clerk**: Takes your personal information, health card, and any insurance information. If you have ever been a patient in that hospital, they can find your hospital file.

    - **Unit clerk:** The centre of information flow, like the "air traffic controller" of the ED. Coordinates paper and phone communication between doctors, nurses, technicians, patients, and their families. Functioning as a switchboard operator, they connect with other parts of the hospital. Must listen and respond to many requests at once.

- **Technicians**

    - **Laboratory tech:** Collects your blood and sends it for analysis. Makes sure the right vials are collected from the right patient.

    - **ECG tech:** Turns your heartbeat into a picture–one of the earliest ways to spot dangers. Doctors might see your ECG before they see your face.

    - **Ortho tech:** Stabilizes body parts such as broken bones or sprained ligaments with casts, splints, or immobilizers.

    - **X-ray tech:** Although they are situated in their own Diagnostic Imaging or Medical Imaging Department, they are called to the ED to do portable X-rays on certain patients that are too sick or unstable to be moved.

- **Respiratory Therapists (RTs)**: Specialize in airway management, devices, and disorders. They keep you breathing. They can also provide coaching on how to use puffers effectively, or give information about oxygen options at home.
- **Porters or unit aides:** Transport patients for tests, to other areas of the hospital, back again to their ED location, or to a hospital ward once admitted. These team members also deliver and restock equipment, and help nurses provide important care to patients, such as helping with personal hygiene and mobilization.
- **Security guards:** Keep everyone safe so we can focus on healthcare. Our workplace can be dangerous when people are agitated and not thinking straight because of drugs, dementia, psychosis, alcohol, infections (we call that *delirium*), or emotional distress. Not only do they protect the staff, but they also protect patients from themselves and self-harm.
- **Learners:** Do real-life training with supervision. You'll see medical, nursing, and paramedic students.

  - **Medical students:** You may be first assessed by a medical student, who is likely in the last half of their schooling. After two years of learning from books, small groups, and cadavers, these "doctors in training" start to apply what they've learned. After they gather information from you, they record and organize this information, and present it to the doctor who is supervising them. Sometimes medical students are more thorough and can spend more time with you than the staff physician, who might just briefly confirm some of your history and double-check some physical exam findings.
  - **Residents**: All newly minted M.D.'s must gain further experience as a *resident*, an apprentice doctor who can work a bit more independently, but who still has to be supervised by a staff physician. They are paid a small amount and work semi-autonomously under the supervision of one or more experienced physicians. A senior resident may be responsible for teaching junior residents and medical students.

- **International medical graduates, rural physicians, search-and-rescue technicians, and military medics** regularly do skills training in the ED.

- **Midlevel providers:** In the USA, it would be more common to have *physician assistants (PAs)* and scribes, professionals who work with physicians to provide healthcare. In Canada, we are starting to see more Nurse Practitioners (NPs), who have additional training and independence.
- **Social worker:** Sometimes the issues run deeper than a simple medication or diagnostic test. Social workers may be able to provide resources regarding housing, finances, health insurance coverage, veteran benefits, and addiction recovery options.
- **Housekeeping staff:** Keep the place clean. The ED is full of blood, urine, feces, and other infectious bodily fluids. Without the house-keeping staff, the ED would have to close up shop. These employees are unsung heroes who don't get the thank-you cards they deserve.

Assume at Your Own Risk

There are many *male nurses* and many *female doctors*. Some staff identify as transgendered.

Don't jump to a mistaken conclusion based on gender or age. It still happens surprisingly frequently.

Basic Emergency Department Layout

In EDs around the world, ranging from big university ones to small rural ones, the following is the typical setup I've seen. EDs are mainly designed around the types of emergencies that might need treatment. For this reason, there are many different types of rooms and each one contains different equipment. The triage nurse helps match a patient to the appropriate room. It wouldn't be helpful to have a heart attack patient in the gynecology room or a person with an ankle sprain on a cardiac monitor.

- **Monitored areas**

  - These areas allow us to continuously monitor a patient's vital signs and their general appearance. These rooms are by and large in view of the main nursing area. See the textbox on **page 13** for the monitoring we use in these rooms and what the lines and numbers displayed mean.

- **Non-monitored areas**

  - These include ambulatory care areas, hallways, and fast-track areas. Ambulatory areas are for the "walking wounded"— people who can move in and out of a stretcher when needed, and sit in a separate area when waiting. Hallways are historically the overflow spaces—not because this is the best thing to do, but because we have no choice, and nowhere else to put patients. Fast-track spaces are used for simple and quick problems like sprained ankles.

- **Specialized rooms**

  - Trauma bay (trauma room, resuscitation room)

    - This is probably what readers picture when thinking about the ED. The sickest of the sick are rushed in here. It is kept stocked with life-saving equipment and medications, a cardiac monitor, defibrillator, oxygen, suction, and more. There is at least one bed reserved for patients who need resuscitation, with plenty of space to allow the different members of the ED healthcare team to do their jobs at the same time. There might be a Respiratory Therapist at the head of the bed managing a patient's airway and breathing. Nurses may be on either side placing an IV line to deliver medications and fluids or blood products, while another nurse stands apart to coordinate and record actions. Physicians may be at the foot of the bed directing the team and watching for changes on the vital signs monitor. Larger centres may have an additional trauma room specifically for pediatric patients.

- Isolation rooms:

  - These negative pressure rooms allow airflow to go only one way: from the main area into the room, but not vice-versa. This helps to keep airborne infectious diseases such as tuberculosis, chickenpox, and measles in the isolation room.

- Eye, Ear, Nose, and Throat (ENT) rooms

  - These rooms have specialized instruments to examine eyes under magnification, to treat a major nosebleed, or to remove a foreign body like a bead up the nose of a child, for example.

- Gyne rooms

  - These rooms contain a stretcher that can be converted to do an internal pelvic exam. They also have lighting that can be adjusted and all the necessary equipment for these types of exams.

- Ortho / cast rooms

  - These rooms contain the equipment needed to make and apply casts and splints.

- Procedure rooms

  - These rooms have more space and better lighting, needed to suture bad cuts and drain abscesses (infected fluid collections).

- Psychiatric rooms

  - There may be a special area to look after people with mental health concerns. These areas may have extra privacy for sensitive conversations. The furniture is also designed to protect the patient from hurting themselves, other patients, or the staff.

- Family / quiet rooms

  - These are quiet and private spaces used to deliver difficult or distressing news about a patient. They allow multiple family members space and time to think and feel whatever they need to. When I have to deliver bad news, these rooms let families honestly express their surprise, grief, anger, confusion, and fear of the unknown.

- Workspaces

  - Doctors and nurses have to document everything that happens during an ED visit, including what medications are given and when. Pen and paper methods are slowly changing to electronic charting using computers and voice dictation microphones. It might seem like they spend more time in front of a screen than in front of patients.

PART 4
ARMCHAIR EMERG DOC

The Internet Will See You Now

It's a common phenomenon now: I search the Internet before I buy a car, try to fix an appliance, mend clothing, or choose a restaurant. Chances are you consult "Dr. Google" when your body is acting up. Many times, it's great for me if you know a little bit about what you might have and the medical jargon we use. In my experience, however, the top results from Internet searches don't always point people to the exceptionally useful and reliable sites.

This section will give you a brief sample of the life-threatening conditions that your medical team is looking for, what your symptoms might suggest, plus some resources I regularly give to patients when I discharge them. Beware of playing "armchair emerg doc" because, as the saying goes, "A little knowledge is a dangerous thing!"

My intention here is to satisfy some of your curiosity, share some tips I've learned over the years, and suggest other sources to learn more. These topics are meant to provide general information only, and this book is not a substitute for speaking to a medical practitioner.

Medical Student Syndrome

A common phenomenon that occurs when a student (medical, dental, nursing) learns enough information to think a disease might apply to themselves!

For example, when I was a 20-something-year-old medical student, I had an episode of chest heaviness. I arrived at the nearest walk-in clinic worried and left humbled. I was not, in fact, having a heart attack—I likely just had heartburn!

Time-sensitive Conditions

As an ED doctor, I'm primarily trying to rule out serious disease. This can be challenging, especially if it's an uncommon condition, or if patients show up with symptoms that aren't typical for a given disease. Unfortunately, we're not always good at giving a label or diagnosis to someone's pain, even after our many tests. Often, I find myself sending a person home with a "label" of chest or abdominal pain NYD (which stands for "Not Yet Diagnosed"), with a recommendation for them to follow up with another physician.

Patients who are about to die tend to be quiet, not loud. The entire department can be preoccupied trying to save someone on the brink of death, yet it wouldn't be obvious to someone waiting down the hall.

Here are just a few of the things we think and worry about, even in people who may not look very sick at first. These can be critical emergencies, and be life or limb-threatening, especially if diagnosed late. The tricky part is that the majority of people that come to the ED with similar symptoms *do not*, in fact, have these dangerous conditions. It's our job to try to tell the difference. A person experiencing these symptoms should always come to the ED and leave it to the physicians to determine what it could be.

Symptoms: Sudden severe pain from the chest or abdomen through to the back

What we worry about: Aortic catastrophes – Your aorta is your body's main "plumbing"—the big blood vessel that carries blood from your heart to the rest of your body. Sometimes it starts to rip apart and cut through the layers of tissue that normally contain all that blood under high pressure.

Symptoms: Severe pain from the chest through to the upper back

What we worry about: Thoracic aortic catastrophe – When the thoracic (chest) section of the aorta is affected, the symptom is classically severe pain felt from the centre of the chest through to the upper back. We believe it is caused by years of high blood pressure, but some conditions (such as *Marfan syndrome* and *Ehlers-Danlos syndrome*) put younger people at risk.

Symptoms: Sudden severe pain from the belly through the back

What we worry about: *Abdominal aortic aneurysm* (AAA) – This occurs when the abdominal section of the aorta ruptures. These usually occur after age 50. The pain is ordinarily felt from the middle of the belly and radiates through to the middle of the back (and not just one side, like with kidney stones). Like a ticking time-bomb, the aneurysm itself is actually silent and slow-growing at first, until it's so big that the bomb goes off. Normally your aorta would measure about 3 cm across. As it bulges over 5 cm, the risk of sudden rupture and death by internal bleeding increases. Once it ruptures, the risk of dying from it may be as high as 90%! If the emergency doctor can diagnose these early, patients can sometimes make it in time for emergency surgery or other treatments.

BEWARE of sudden, very severe pain in the front of the chest or abdomen that shoots through to the middle of the back. The pain is characteristically constant and doesn't get better or worse with movement, rest, position, activity, meals, or breathing. Narcotic medications like morphine may not even help.

Symptoms: Ongoing chest pain or heaviness

What we worry about: Heart attack a.k.a. *myocardial infarction* (MI) – Many people think of our classic patient as someone arriving at the ED, clutching at their chest, having a heart attack. However, some people can have a heart attack without pain. This is more common in people with diabetes, for example. Women and the elderly may not have the "textbook" signs and symptoms.

BEWARE of ongoing chest pain, heaviness, or discomfort that lasts for at least minutes (not just seconds), especially if severe and/or there is also:

- Pain spreading to the arms, neck, or jaw
- Sweating
- Shortness of breath

Symptoms: Sudden weakness of one side of the body, changes in speech, or drooping of part of the face

What we worry about: Stroke a.k.a. *cerebrovascular accident* (CVA) – Sometimes a stroke is obvious—the person suddenly can't move one side of their body, or their speech is slurred, or there is a sudden change in their face, such as one side drooping. Sometimes this is caused by a clot in a blood vessel, though sometimes it is caused by a blood vessel that ruptures and bleeds. Both can cause serious damage to the brain, but the treatments for clotting versus bleeding are very different. If we can catch a severe stroke early enough, there are new ways to grab the clot to allow blood to flow again to the brain. For this reason, it's crucially important to recognize symptoms of a stroke and to get to the ED immediately.

BEWARE of sudden…

- **Numbness or weakness** in the face, arm, or leg, especially on one side of the body
- **Confusion**, trouble speaking, or difficulty understanding speech
- **Trouble seeing** in one or both eyes
- **Trouble walking** or loss of balance
- **Lack of coordination** such as being unable to write or use a phone
- **Severe "worst-ever" headache** with no known cause

Call 9-1-1 right away if you or someone else has any of these symptoms.

How to Tell if Someone May Be Having a Stroke

F—Face: Ask the person to smile. Does one side of the face droop?

A—Arms: Ask the person to raise both arms. Does one arm drift downward?

S—Speech: Ask the person to repeat a simple phrase. Is the speech slurred or strange?

T—Time: If you see any of these signs, call 9-1-1 **right away.**

Symptoms: Loss of vision in one eye

What we worry about: Retinal detachment – This is a problem that can cause permanent blindness. We try to catch people with these visual symptoms early so we can refer them to an ophthalmologist for emergency treatment.

BEWARE of:

- Many tiny "**floaters**" or black spots when looking through one eye, or **flashes of lights or bright spots**. These are occasionally the first signs of a retinal detachment.
- Any **new painless loss of vision in one eye**, especially if it's as if a "**curtain**" has pulled across part of your visual field (such as your side vision).

Symptoms: Lower abdominal pain and/or vaginal bleeding

What we worry about: *Ectopic pregnancy* – Sometimes a fertilized egg ends up in the wrong place instead of in the womb. As the fertilized egg grows, it can rupture and cause internal bleeding that can actually threaten a woman's life. For example, in a tubal pregnancy, the growing mass is in the area of the Fallopian tube on one side. The woman may or may not even know that she's even pregnant. The bleeding can seem like an early miscarriage.

BEWARE of **pain** in the lower abdomen and/or vaginal **bleeding during early pregnancy.**

Symptoms: Fever plus fainting, or persistent confusion/drowsiness

What we worry about: Sepsis – A bad infection can get into the bloodstream and cause low blood pressure, causing what we call "septic shock." This can cause multi-organ failure. Patients with sepsis need antibiotics quickly, and IV fluids are essential.

BEWARE of **fever plus fainting** (caused by low blood pressure), persistent **confusion**, or **drowsiness**.

Worrisome to Patients, But Not an Emergency After All

This is not a substitute for medical advice and, if in doubt, readers should call a nurse/family doctor for advice.

High Blood Pressure by Itself

Normal blood pressure is less than 120/80. It's surprisingly common for people to come to the Emergency worried after discovering a high blood pressure reading. Sometimes they've taken their blood pressure using a machine at the pharmacy or grocery store. Other times, they may have a home blood pressure machine and be alarmed by a significant rise in their numbers compared to what they're used to seeing.

By itself, high blood pressure—even with numbers such as 200/160—is *not* an emergency when there are no other symptoms. For people who come into the ED worried about high blood pressure, we tend to do blood tests, but these tests are almost always normal, and we often send the patients home with no new medications.

Why is that?

- High blood pressure *does* put you at risk of developing heart disease and problems in and around the brain. However, that risk builds up over many years to decades. High blood pressure for weeks and even months does not tend to cause problems that require people to need ED treatment.
- High blood pressure is predominantly silent. If someone has not checked their blood pressure in a long time, they wouldn't know that their blood pressure has been at this level for ages. In other words, their health has been the same for weeks and likely will be the same for weeks to come.
- Temporary fluctuations can happen. Blood pressure numbers change minute to minute. If you've had caffeine recently, if you're in pain, or

if you're stressed and worried (about having high blood pressure, for example) then your blood pressure will temporarily rise.

- Falsely high readings. If the blood pressure cuff is too small for your arm, or you haven't been quietly sitting still for several minutes before checking your blood pressure, the numbers you get are likely to be falsely high.
- The first treatments for high blood pressure are primarily lifestyle changes. If your regular doctor measured high blood pressure in the office or clinic, they would ask you to exercise more, eat less salt and processed foods, find ways to manage your stress, and quit smoking. Of course, it takes a while before these lifestyle changes lower blood pressure. So, your doctor would ask you to come back for a recheck down the road. We provide the same advice in the ED.
- Lowering blood pressure too quickly is more likely to cause harm than watchful waiting. When people arrive at the ED with a high blood pressure reading, after they simply sit around and wait for a while, their blood pressure improves ordinarily. Using medications to lower blood pressure very suddenly can *cause* a stroke, dizziness, fainting, and falls.
- We are taught in medicine to "treat the patient, not the monitor." With any blood pressure reading, we need to consider the person's overall health needs more than the actual blood pressure number.

BEWARE: If a person has high blood pressure readings AND any of the following symptoms, it's important to see a medical professional or go to the nearest ED:

- Chest pain, especially if it is severe or moves into the back
- Breathing problems
- Vision changes
- A bad headache
- Repeated vomiting

Eye Complaints

I often see people for eye complaints, as they are understandably worried about their vision. The following two issues don't need much medical attention at all, and you can safely follow up with your primary care doctor if things don't settle down over time.

Stye

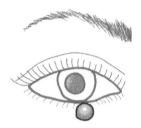

This is basically a pimple in the eyelash area. Would you come to the ED for a zit? It can certainly be very sore and look angry, but all we'll tell you to do is to put a hot (but not scalding) moist cloth on the area frequently (10 minutes, four times a day, for a few days). This will help the pus come to a head and, eventually, it will drain on its own. Don't try to "pop" a stye. Wash your hands before and after you apply the cloth to the stye, and try to keep your hands away from your eyes (a good idea all the time, by the way).

Subconjuctival hemorrhage

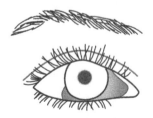

This is the medical term for a burst blood vessel on the surface of the eye that is normally white (the *sclera*). It can look very dramatic! Classically, the area of redness appears suddenly, only affects the white of the eye (not the coloured part—the *iris*), affects only one eye, and is painless. Because it causes minimal to no symptoms, you may have only noticed it in the mirror or when someone else pointed it out to you. If your eye wasn't recently injured in some way, and your eye looks similar to this photo, you don't need to lose any sleep over it. The treatment is just time; it will slowly resolve on its own, typically after one to two weeks. A colleague of mine points out to his patients that if this was anywhere else on your body it would look like a small bruise—and he advises that they don't need to be any more concerned about it than a bruise on their arm.

Tips on Using Eye Drops

Do you blink every time you try to put in eye drops? Ever struggled to put drops in your squirming child's eye?

Here's an easy and non-traumatic way to get those drops in:

- Get the eye drop bottle ready.

- Have the person lie down and *close* their eyes.

- Place a drop in the corner (the corner closest to the nose) of their *closed* eye. There is a small well that is formed by the two eyelids and the bridge of the nose.

- While they are still lying down, ask the person to open their eyes and blink a few times.

Presto! The drop follows gravity and bathes the surface of the eye. Now repeat with the other eye if needed!

You can modify this technique to put drops in *your own eye*, too. By laying down and keeping one eye open, you can try to place a drop near the corner of your closed eye. Just keep some tissue or a cloth handy in case your aim is off.

Your Symptoms and What They Might Mean

The human body is amazing and complex. One of the hard parts about my job as an emergency physician is being comfortable with the unknown. Nearly all of the people we see are people we know nothing about. Sometimes—even after all our acute care tests—we can't figure out the cause of a person's presenting concern. Certainly, we learn common patterns that allow us to help many patients, but everybody (and *every body*) is different. There are exceptions to every pattern.

For example, someone may come in complaining of pain on the lower right-hand side of their abdominal area. They tell us the pain is constant and getting worse. What could this be? Possibly appendicitis. But other possible diagnoses may include diverticulitis; a kidney stone that is trying to pass but is getting stuck; an ovary that is twisted on itself and strangulating; Crohn's disease or another form of colitis; constipation; cancer that's been growing silently until now; a hernia that's pushing through the muscle layer that normally holds your bowels in place… and potentially a dozen more things. This list of possible causes is what we call a "Differential Diagnosis" list or DDx for short.

When to Suspect Appendicitis

The classic location of appendicitis pain is a spot known as *McBurney's point*.

To find it…

- Put your hands on your hips.

- With your right index finger, you should feel a prominent rounded edge of your hip bone.

- Draw an imaginary line between that spot to your belly button.

- About one-third of the way along that line is where *McBurney's point* lies.

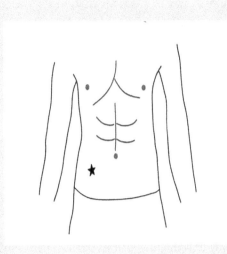

If you have abdominal pain that is constant but has moved to that Point, and it's tender if you press there, I would be worried about appendicitis. Time to go to the ED!

Pain

If you can provide the following details it will help your ED team try to figure out the cause of your pain. When we take a history of any patient's pain, we use this helpful memory aid—OPQRST—to make sure we get all the important information.

OPQRST

Onset – Did the pain begin suddenly or gradually?

Precipitating and relieving factors – What makes the pain better/worse? Certain positions or movements, for example? What about if you eat food or take over-the-counter pain medications?

Quality – A description of the pain, which can be difficult. Is it sharp or dull? Electric or burning? Crampy? A tightness? Can you pinpoint it to one spot, or is it vague and spread out?

Radiation – Does the pain stay in a certain spot, or do you feel it elsewhere? For example, abdominal pain can shoot through to the back or up to the shoulder tip. Back pain can shoot down to the knee or all the way to the toes.

Severity – Mild, medium, or severe ranking out of 10, with 10 being the worst pain you can imagine. Did it start out terrible and then ease off, or progress to a maximum level you are currently at?

Timing – Was there something that happened right before the pain began? Do you still have pain? If it comes and goes, is the pain there for seconds, minutes, or hours at a time?

Fever

Fever is your body's way of signalling that its defence mechanisms are kicking in. Usually, fever is a sign of an infection; however, the infection might be due to something mild (such as a "cold" virus) or something more severe, such as a bacterial infection. If the infection is caused by a common virus, your body often fights it on its own. Antibiotics will only help if the infection is caused by bacteria.

Why do doctors recommend antipyretic (anti-fever) medications such as acetaminophen and ibuprofen? Because you'll tend to feel lousy with a fever—in addition to feeling hot and unwell, you may have pain, chills, or sweats. These medications can help you feel less uncomfortable. They don't treat the underlying cause of the fever or help us figure out what's causing the fever. Feel free to take something so you aren't suffering! However, as with all medications, don't take more than the recommended dose on the bottle, and check with a pharmacist if you are taking multiple medications, prescription or otherwise (See Home Medicine Cabinet, page 72)

BEWARE: We worry about a fever when...

- There is also fainting, ongoing drowsiness, or confusion
- There is also a headache and stiff neck
- You are vomiting so badly that pills and sips won't stay down
- You have a seizure
- A rash appears
- You're not fully vaccinated

- You've recently travelled abroad
- The fever lasts more than five days

If you experience any of these plus fever, seek urgent medical attention through your regular doctor's clinic or go to the ED.

MYTH: Don't take medications before you see a doctor because it might "mask" the fever or pain

FACT: Whether you have a low-grade fever or a more pronounced temperature is less important than the context you have the fever in. We will make decisions more on your health status and risks and what we are worried about, not so much on the exact number. So go ahead and take those over-the-counter medications. Otherwise, we will be using the same ones as first-line agents before advancing to stronger ones.

FACT: Some people don't have a fever even when they have a serious infection. So, we can't rely on just the temperature reading, especially for populations including newborns, the elderly, the immunocompromised, and those with diabetes.

FACT: Doctors used to avoid giving pain relief to patients with abdominal pain for fear that it would "mask" appendicitis or other cases that would need surgery. We've changed our minds because the examination and findings were shown by research studies to actually be MORE accurate after some pain control was given. It might be time to change your mind, too.

Home Medicine Cabinet

It's amazing how many people wait hours in the ED *without* having tried anything at home first! If they have, often it's not necessarily the best medication or at the right dose and frequency. One of the benefits of medical school training is learning simple, cheap, and effective medications for common ailments. But it doesn't take four years of medical school to learn.

The confusing thing is that there are at least two different names for every medication: the generic name and the brand/trade name.

The best way to know what's in the over-the-counter (OTC) medications (those you can buy without a prescription) is to check the small print on the side or back of the packaging that lists the "active medical ingredients."

There are dozens of boxes and bottles in those rows at the food and drug store. But these are often variations of the same medication. Brand name pills in different flavors and formulations sit next to generic or "store brand" ones. Manufacturers create combination drugs that have two or three different active ingredients in one convenient tablet or capsule.

Speak to a pharmacist if you are starting a new medication, are already on medications, or have questions about a particular medication.

How Do I Choose What Medication to Buy Over the Counter?

I am a cost-conscious consumer so I mainly buy the generic versions of all medications when I can. There are certain formulations that don't have an equivalent yet, such as a long-acting version, or a rapidly dissolving version, so I might buy those branded ones if I needed them.

I also check how many milligrams ("mg") are contained in each pill and the number of pills in each package. Then I choose the box or bottle that gives me the greatest amount of medication for the lowest price.

Personally, I prefer to avoid combination pills that have multiple active ingredients so I can maximize the effectiveness of each medication for the purpose I want.

Medications Everyone Should Have

The following medications are readily available at pharmacies and grocery stores. However, I would recommend having them all at home in advance, stored in a safe area. When someone is feeling unwell enough to need these medications, they do not want to be waiting in a shopping lineup.

*Typical adult dose

** Always read and follow the instructions on the label! People with some conditions such as diabetes, kidney disease, bleeding disorders, or specific drug allergies must be careful about taking any over-the-counter medicines. Read labels closely and be sure to ask your doctor or pharmacist if you have any questions.

Generic name	Brand Name	Use	Why	Dose*	Cautions**
Acetaminophen	Tylenol	Aches, pain, and fever	Likely the safest medication we have for pain	Up to 1000 mg per dose, up to 4 times a day	Be careful if taking other pain or cold medications, as they are often combined with acetaminophen. Check the back of the package under "medicinal ingredients"
ASA (acetylsalicylic acid)	Aspirin	For suspected heart attack	If someone, even a guest, is having chest pain, 9-1-1 may advise this medication be given	80-325 mg, likely to be chewed	I don't recommend it for pain and fever because it can affect bleeding and clotting
Ibuprofen	Advil / Motrin	Aches, pain, and fever	Works better as an anti-inflammatory, and lasts longer than acetaminophen	Up to 400 mg per dose, up to 4 times a day	Avoid if you have a history of diabetes, kidney problems, confirmed ulcers, or bleeding problems
Hydrocortisone cream		Localized itch / swelling	A gentle anti-inflammatory that can be combined with allergy pills	Rub in twice a day	Most useful for small areas
Diphenhydramine	Benadryl	Itch / allergic reaction	Works quickly	25-50 mg per dose, every 4-6 hours	May cause drowsiness. Do not drive or do anything where you need your wits about you
Cetirizine / Loratadine / Desloratadine	Reactine / Claritin / Aerius	Itch / allergic reaction	Non-drowsy, long-acting. Very safe even at double dose, and can be combined with other medications. Even children can take a regular adult dissolvable dose ("rapid-melt") if they can't swallow pills	1-2 tablets daily (0.5-1 tablet daily for children)	May be slower to work than Benadryl. Not to be used on its own for serious allergy/anaphylaxis.

Dimenhydrinate	Gravol	Nausea and vomiting	Helpful to have around because when vomiting strikes it can be hard to rush out to the store (if it's even open)	25-50 mg per dose, every 4-6 hours. Or 1-2 children's chewable if difficulty with swallowing pills or keeping them down	Often causes drowsiness—do not drive or do anything where you need your wits about you
Xylometazoline nasal spray/drops	Otrivin	Nasal congestion and more	Can also be used for nosebleeds that keep starting up	1 or 2 sprays / drops into each nostril, every 8-10 hours	See page 99 - 100 for tips on how to use. Do not use for more than 5 days before taking a few days off. Otherwise, if you use it for a long continuous period, there is a rebound effect where your symptoms will come back with a vengeance when you stop it.
Loperamide	Imodium	Diarrhea	Slows down your bowels	4 mg at first, with repeat doses of 2 mg as needed	There's a saying, "better out than in…" as in, your body may be trying to empty itself of something in your digestive system. I would aim to just decrease how many trips to the bathroom you make, rather than trying to fully return to normal

Pain medications do come in liquid form, but when a child gets big enough they need a lot of liquid to get an adequate dose of medication—sometimes more than they want to swallow despite how sweet the manufacturers make it. For my three kids, I always had at home children's **chewable** medications for pain and fever. The doses we use in the ED are: 10 mg/kg (to a maximum of 400 mg) per dose of ibuprofen, and 15 mg/kg (to a maximum of 500 mg) per dose for acetaminophen. However, there is a risk of miscalculation here, so I suggest double-checking with a pharmacist or medical professional before doing this for ages or weights not listed on the package of chewable medication.

Medication Safety

Name Alert!

Note the similarities between the generic names *di***phen***hydram***INE** and *di***men***hydrin***ATE**. To help you remember the difference, think of the –ATE ending at the end of dimenhydrinate as relating to the stomach (nausea). Other similar-looking names might be **aceta***minophen* and **acetyl***salicylic acid (ASA).*

Your Friendly Neighborhood Pharmacist

Your local pharmacist can…

- Recommend which medications and over-the-counter treatments might be beneficial for you. This is especially true if you are taking many prescriptions, as they are aware of the possible interactions between drugs that can happen.

  Common conditions that may have an over-the-counter treatment include lice, warts, hemorrhoids, vaginal yeast infections, diarrhea or constipation, irritable bowel syndrome, seasonal allergies, pinworms, and itchy skin.

- Talk to you about your prescription medications. If you wish to stop a prescription, they can advise which ones are more likely to cause side effects if stopped suddenly. Some medications are best stopped by gradually reducing the dose over a period of time.

- Prescribe a limited number of medications. This varies greatly by province.

- Properly dispose of unwanted or unused medications. Your pharmacy can safely discard them. Never flush them down the toilet! They can contaminate our water sources.

What About Expiration Dates?

Unlike milk that goes sour quickly, or nuts that turn rancid, medications don't tend to go bad the same way. They are unlikely to turn dangerous or toxic after they've been sitting on the shelf too long. What is probable to happen is that they become slightly less potent after a long period of time.

"Most of what is known about drug expiration dates comes from a study conducted by the Food and Drug Administration at the request of the military. With a large and expensive stockpile of drugs, the military faced tossing out and replacing its drugs every few years. (What they found from the study is 90% of more than 100 drugs, both prescription and over-the-counter, were perfectly good to use even 15 years after the expiration date."[7]

A British Antarctic Survey study "suggests that certain drugs, up to 51 months post-expiry … appear to be stable with no significant breakdown products."[8]

Prevent Medication Overdoses!

Accidental drug overdoses are one of the leading causes of death. Even seemingly common medications such as Aspirin (ASA) or Tylenol (acetaminophen) can be toxic in high doses.

- Keep **all medications** up high, out of reach, and out of sight to prevent kids of all ages from swallowing something they shouldn't.

- Be extra careful how you store **narcotics** (opioid pain medications). Sadly, many teens become addicted to these pain relievers after discovering them in their parents' or grandparents' medicine cabinets.

---

7   Harvard Health Publishing. *"Drug Expiration Dates—Do They Mean Anything?"* Last modified Dec 13, 2019. *https://www.health.harvard.edu/staying-healthy/drug-expiration-dates-do-they-mean-anything.*

8   Browne E. "Expired Drugs in the Remote Environment," *Wilderness & Environmental Medicine* 30, 1 (2019): 28-34. https://doi.org/10.1016/j.wem.2018.11.003.

- If you have opioids in your house, ask your pharmacist for a free **home naloxone kit** in case you ever have to treat someone if you suspect an opioid overdose. This could save their life.

- Put the telephone for your local **Poison Control Centre** in your phone's contacts and have it written down beside your landline.

What Doesn't Work?

Many products out there have limited or no evidence that they actually help. Certainly, some people benefit from the placebo effect. Personally, I'd rather not waste my money on something that's unlikely to make a difference.

Cough Syrups

I still cringe at the memory of artificial cherry or grape-flavored syrup I was made to take as a kid; in hindsight, these medicines probably did me almost no good. Most coughs and "colds" are due to one of several different viruses that we don't have an effective treatment for. Because antibiotics are only useful for bacterial infections (like antifungals are only useful for fungal infections), they are also unhelpful for these types of viral respiratory tract infections.

Instead, try honey for children over age one. Evidence suggests honey probably relieves cough severity and shortens duration compared to placebo or doing nothing.[9]

Herbal Supplements and Detoxes

I also cringe thinking of the millions of dollars spent each year on herbal supplements and "detoxes" that might have no proven benefit but do have documented evidence of harm.[10]

---

9   Oduwole O., Udoh E. E. "Honey for acute cough in children," *Cochrane Database of Systematic Reviews* (2018): Issue 4. DOI: 10.1002/14651858.CD007094.pub5.

10   Cohen P. A. "Emergency department visits and hospitalisations for adverse events related to dietary supplements are common," *BMJ Evidence-Based Medicine,* 21 (2016): 79.

Despite advertising and packaging, studies in fact mostly fail to show any improvement.[11] In the USA, an estimated 23,000 ED visits per year are attributed to adverse events related to dietary supplements.[12]

In Canada, pharmaceutical companies can sell products to treat and cure medical conditions, but are not allowed to advertise their products directly to the public; yet the companies that make and market Natural Health Products are allowed to market their products directly to Canadians, though they are not allowed to claim that their products can be used to treat or cure a medical condition. However, an independent non-profit consumer protection watchdog and science advocacy organization found, alarmingly, that it was very common for online retailers to ignore Health Canada Regulations. In their report, these retailers frequently made direct and indirect claims that their products can cure medical conditions such as cancer.[13]

11   Office of Dietary Supplements. "Evidence Based Review Program," National Institutes of Health. USA. Accessed July, 2020. https://ods.od.nih.gov/Research/Evidence-Based_Review_Program.aspx.

12   Geller, A. "Emergency Department Visits for Adverse Events Related to Dietary Supplements," *New England Journal of Medicine,* 373. (2015): 1531-1540. DOI: 10.1056/NEJMsa1504267.

13   Bad Science Watch. "NHP Marketing in Canada: A Survey of the Online Marketing of Natural Health Products for Cancer Treatment and Cure," Accessed July, 2020. https://badsciencewatch.ca/natural-health-product-retailers-sell-cancer-cures.

The Life of a Typical Viral Infection

It's helpful to know how a typical viral infection plays out and how your body's internal defences respond. When you catch a virus, it starts making millions of copies of itself (*replicates*), and the more copies it makes, the worse you feel. The worst symptoms often occur three to five days after infection. As your body's immune system kicks in you may have a fever, making you feel hot and cold, with sweats and chills.

Key points:

- In the first few days of illness, bacterial infections and viral infections in the average healthy person can be hard to tell apart—for both the patient and the doctor.
- Signs that might cause us to worry, including hearing noisy lung sounds with a stethoscope, or an abnormal chest X-ray, may not be present right away. We ordinarily need you to have been sick for longer before we can start figuring out what is wrong. For a majority of healthy adults that show up in the first 24-48 hours, when the illness is mild and hasn't progressed rapidly, there is little we can do to help you feel better other than simple over-the-counter medications suggested in "Medications Everyone Should Have" (see page **72**).
- Exceptions to this would include, but are not limited to, if you have underlying heart or lung disease, diabetes, immune suppression, or a chronic medical condition.
- The replicating virus tries to spread itself by making your saliva and mucous ("snot") contagious. You can help prevent the spread of small particles that might make people around you sick by covering your mouth when you cough/sneeze, washing your hands frequently, and disposing of tissue paper carefully in a closed container. When you come to the hospital, you bring those infectious secretions to people who are frail or have weakened immunity.

- The post-viral cough (the "tickle reflex," as I call it) is a periodic after-effect of the irritation and inflammation caused by the virus. It can cause an annoying cough that can last for up to six weeks after a common cold. This continued hacking cough that is slow to disappear is very bothersome, but often not a medically significant concern unless it is accompanied by other problems such as a fever that comes back again, shortness of breath, chest pain, or worsening symptoms.

Tips and Tricks for Common Conditions

Allergic Reaction

Simple hives by and large aren't more than a nuisance. Cool wet cloths or an ice pack can help the itch. Antihistamines available over-the-counter can help them settle down (See page 72, "Home Medicine Cabinet").

Serious allergic reactions classically occur *quickly* after the exposure, and with *more symptoms* that can be severe or widespread. Major reactions can include swelling of the lips, mouth, or tongue. Airway tightening and swelling can cause difficulty breathing, or wheezing, and a drop in blood pressure can cause light-headedness or even fainting. Call 9-1-1 if you have any of these symptoms. Ambulances will have epinephrine to treat possible anaphylaxis. So will pharmacies, doctor's offices, and public health clinics if you happen to be next to one.

If you or a family member have a history of anaphylaxis or severe allergy, here are some key recommendations:

- Get and wear a bracelet or necklace that identifies your allergy in case you are unable to speak (brand names include "Medic-Alert").
- Have an auto-injector of epinephrine (a.k.a. adrenaline, brand names Epi-Pen or Twin-Ject) with you *at all times*, and ideally, a spare that other people can quickly find if needed. This is the most important medication to use for severe allergic reactions.
  - You should always have a current injector (one that has not expired) handy. However, an old expired injector is likely still good, as long as the liquid isn't cloudy. In a severe reaction, getting an injection with medication that's been sitting on the shelf for a long time is still better than no injection.

- Know which end is the needle, so you don't accidentally inject your thumb. To be extra careful, never hold your thumb on top when grasping the auto-injector.
- The medication absorbs fastest when injected in the outer mid-thigh. Another location is the deltoid muscle, which is on the outer side of your shoulder, a few finger widths below the bony part.

- Tape a box of antihistamine tablets to your epinephrine package or the injector itself.

  - An antihistamine is safe to take at the first sign of a mild or moderate allergic reaction, even if you're not sure if the epinephrine is needed.
  - Chewing the medication will make it absorb even faster, but it may taste bitter and powdery.
  - The children's chewable version tastes better, but is a lower dose, so adults may need more (conventionally 50 mg worth).
  - Anti-allergy medications are safe to take in combination with the injected epinephrine, but they are not a good substitute when having major reactions because they can take longer to start working.

- If you also have an underlying lung disease such as asthma or chronic obstructive pulmonary disease (COPD), then an anaphylactic reaction can be riskier to your breathing. Be sure to have a fast-acting inhaler (such as salbutamol, "Ventolin") with you, and perhaps a backup with your Allergic Reaction Toolkit (see the sidebar).

- An oral steroid such as Prednisone or Dexamethasone can be very helpful in reducing swelling and spasm for moderate and severe reactions. It's one of the first medications we give in the ED. However, it can take hours to reach its maximum effect. If you get bad reactions regularly and have needed prescription steroids before, consider asking your doctor for an extra dose to start at the first sign of trouble.

> ### Your Allergic Reaction Toolkit
>
> - **Epi-Pen** (auto-injector of epinephrine)
> - **Anti-Allergy Pills:**
>   - Benadryl (fast-acting)
>   - Claritin, Aerius, Reactine (long-acting)
> - **Asthma medications:**
>   - Fast-acting inhaler (such as salbutamol/Ventolin)
> - **Hydrocortisone cream** (for small areas of itching/hives)
> - **Prescription oral steroid** (for select patients)

Back Pain

Back pain is a very common reason for people to come to the ED. We call it "soft-tissue" or "mechanical" back pain when it comes from the muscles, ligaments, discs, plus the inflammation that surrounds all of those things. Often, people have a history of a minor injury and similar mild episodes of back pain that have gotten better without needing an emergency visit. But sometimes, bending, lifting, or twisting will aggravate an old injury into a bad flare-up. Sometimes the pain is so terrible that it's hard to walk. Other times, pain or numbness and tingling can shoot all the way down the leg to the foot because of nerves that travel from the back to the legs. We call this *sciatica*.

Unfortunately, mechanical back pain can be stubborn to treat. Also, for most people, testing to find the precise cause and location doesn't actually help lessen their pain. In fact, we are trying to reduce the waste of money and time spent across North America on over-investigation of early back pain. (See the sidebar.) For example, even though people want to know if the source of the problem is a disc bulge, knowing the exact source doesn't change the treatment. Frustratingly, we don't have one really effective treatment that doesn't come with side effects, and surgery is rarely the answer. Generally, treatment consists of attempting a number of different possible solutions to improve how well a person can move, and reduce their symptoms a little bit. It's unlikely that any one thing will bring the pain down to zero, but we hope that something or a combination of things will work well enough to get you moving well again in time. The realistic time frame for how long to expect the pain to last is weeks rather than days.

Choosing Wisely

Starting in 2012, medical societies and foundations teamed up with Consumer Reports to identify five tests and treatments, for multiple specialities, that were overused and did not provide meaningful benefit for patients. These have been compiled and communicated under the Choosing Wisely campaign for making evidence-based health decisions. This has become a global movement that now spans over 20 countries.

See https://www.choosingwisely.org/patient-resources and

https://choosingwiselycanada.org/patient-pamphlets

For back pain:

"Back pain can be excruciating. So it seems that getting an X-ray, CT scan, or MRI to find the cause would be a good idea. But that's usually not the case. Here's why:

• They don't help you get better faster.

Most people with lower back pain feel better in about a month whether they get an imaging test or not. In fact, those tests can lead to additional procedures that complicate recovery. For example, one large study of people with back pain found that those who had imaging tests soon after reporting the problem fared no better and sometimes did worse than people who took simple steps like applying heat, staying active, and taking an over-the-counter (OTC) pain reliever. Another study found that back pain sufferers who had an MRI in the first month were eight times more likely to have surgery, but didn't recover faster.

• They can pose risks.

X-rays and CT scans expose you to radiation, which can increase cancer risk. While back x-rays deliver less radiation, they still can give 75 times more radiation than a chest x-ray. That's especially worrisome to men and women of child-bearing age because x-rays and CT scans of the lower back can expose testicles and ovaries to radiation. Furthermore, the tests often reveal spinal abnormalities that could be completely unrelated to the pain. Those findings can cause needless worry and lead to unnecessary follow-up tests and procedures such as injections or sometimes even surgery."[14]

• Findings are not often specific to your pain.

Degenerative disc disease (arthritic changes) and disc bulges can often be found at multiple levels in your spine. If you had an MRI before the pain started, it's possible the same imaging changes would already have been seen and you would not have noticed any symptoms. The changes happen slowly over time.

A disc herniation can return to normal in time. If you have an imaging test too early, it might show something that doesn't change the initial treatment plan, and might be resolved on an imaging test done later on. Disc bulges are not necessarily permanent conditions, but rather, they can resorb back to where they were, or dissolve, months later.

I've had back pain come and go over the years. It seems to return much more often than I'd like and can be really hard to get rid of. I enjoy a massage when my back acts up, especially when combined with heat, mindful breathing, and purposefully trying to relax the muscles that are in spasm. Plus, I've learned to avoid things that tend to make it flare up and I have found some things that help mine settle down in days instead of months.

Here are *10 tips* you may not have tried to help manage the pain and disability of run-of-the-mill back pain:

---

14 "Imaging Tests for Lower Back Pain: When You Need Them and When You Don't." Choosing Wisely Canada, September 17, 2019. https://choosingwiselycanada.org/imaging-tests-low-back-pain.

1) **Heat**. A hot-water bottle or a microwaveable bean bag can bring some temporary relief. After you apply some heat, you may find it a good time to stretch and gain some more range of motion.

2) **Anti-inflammatories**. See the section on Medications Everyone Should Have at Home (**page 72**) for more information on who should and shouldn't use over-the-counter medications such as ibuprofen. Prescription anti-inflammatories aren't necessarily any better or stronger, sometimes they are just more convenient because they can be taken once a day. You could also try a medicated rub such as diclofenac (Brand Name: Voltaren) that delivers the pain medication directly to the area that hurts.

3) **Self-massage.** I found certain massage therapists to be helpful, and I even tried buying an automatic massage chair when my back acted up. But not everyone can access these, nor is there strong evidence of benefit. There are some simple techniques that involve putting something on the floor, laying on top of it, and rolling around to put pressure on different muscles next to your spine. Try to avoid too much pressure on your bony spine and neck. Experiment with foam rollers of different sizes and firmness. Some people use two tennis balls in a stocking. There are also inflatable versions that allow you to vary the pressure.

4) **Keep moving** as best you can! The worst thing you can do for your back is to stay still, as this can lead to more stiffness, which then leads to more pain, creating a vicious cycle. So, *avoid bed rest*, and don't stay in one position for too long.

5) **Try walking** as much as you can. Aim for at least 20 minutes three times a week and then increase this slowly as you get stronger.

6) **Swim or try walking and stretching underwater**. These are ways to keep moving using the gentle resistance of the water.

7) **TENS** or *Transcutaneous Electrical Nerve Stimulation*. This is a non-invasive therapy that causes a mild pulsing sensation or muscle twitching that may offer some relief of pain. It has been safely used during pregnancy by women for decades. There are consumer models you can buy and learn to use. Avoid placing the stickers on the head or neck area.

8) **Yoga**. Look for gentle classes that use props and guided stretches such as Restorative Yoga or Yoga for Back Care. Tell your instructor about any injured locations or pain that is bothering you.

9) **Physiotherapy**. Different therapists will give you various exercises to try, suggesting which muscles to target. Importantly, they often do a very detailed assessment and may offer treatments including manipulation, massage, and ultrasound.

10) **Acupuncture**. There seems to be some modest evidence for benefit. However, this may vary depending on the acupuncturist delivering the treatment. Be sure to carefully check the credentials and reputation of anyone who offers acupuncture.

BEWARE: Do seek medical attention if you have any of the following with your back pain:

- You suddenly become incontinent (you can't hold your bladder or bowels and start having "accidents"). Note that this isn't ordinarily an emergency if you *already had problems* with this before the back pain, or if it's happening because you can't *get* to the bathroom quickly enough because of this pain.
- Weight loss
- Night sweats or fever and chills
- Numbness down both your legs or in the area of your anus where you would wipe
- "Foot drop" where your foot seems to drag when you walk normally and you can't walk on your heels.
- If your pain started immediately after an impact injury
- You've been diagnosed with cancer before, in the unlikely event it has spread to the bone
- The pain is severe or associated with any pain in the front of your body, such as the chest or abdomen
- Younger patients who have back pain that is *worse after rest*, such as first thing in the morning, and that gets *better with exercise* and activity

Concussion

Minor head injury is a common reason for people to seek medical attention. While an assessment by a medical professional can be helpful, very few people will need diagnostic imaging tests.

A concussion is a brain injury caused by *blunt trauma*, such as a fall, or a blow to the head. Sometimes these injuries are very severe and we can see swelling or blood when we do imaging tests. However, we think concussions are the result of microscopic injury to the brain that *doesn't* show up on our standard imaging tests.

Prevalent symptoms of concussion include headache, nausea, loss of concentration or focus, and feeling "off."

Some things likely make concussion symptoms better:

- **Physical rest**. Avoid exercise and sports until you are feeling back to normal. Rest as if you had the stomach flu and were taking it easy at home.
- **Sleep**. Once upon a time, we used to recommend waking people in the middle of the night. We no longer recommend this. In fact, resting the brain and body are some of the key steps in recovery.
- **Mental rest**. Make sure your environment is quiet and dim (low lighting). Reduce stimulation such as reading, watching television, or using screens such as computers and phones. Avoid tasks (as much as you can) that require focus, concentration, and a lot of brainpower.
- **Hydration**. Drink plenty of fluids, but avoid caffeine and alcohol.

Don't try to rush your recovery. We suggest a graduated, step-wise return to activity:

- *After* your symptoms normalize, once you feel more like yourself, you can start doing a little bit more at a time. For example, if after a day of rest, you have no headache, nausea, or disorientation, try a little bit of gentle activity around the home. The next day, if you feel just as well, you could try going for a short and gentle walk. After that, you can gradually increase the time and strenuousness of activity each day.

- Add in non-contact practice and sports, before trying to return to any regular activities that are more intense.
- If you can, take some time off work or school and any activities that require a lot of thinking, concentration, and focus. Schedule breaks to ease back into your routine. Giving yourself a chance to heal at the beginning may ultimately help speed your return to normal in the long run.
- If, at any point, symptoms return, then your body is telling you that you're doing too much too soon! Back off the physical activities or mental tasks, and rest more.

BEWARE: Go to the ED if you have any of the following with your head injury:

- You're taking any blood thinners that are stronger than aspirin (ASA).
- Repeated episodes of vomiting.
- Severe headache, especially sudden and worst-ever.
- Vision or speech loss, or the inability to use your arm or leg.
- You are so drowsy that it's hard to wake up or get up during times of day when you would normally be awake.

What can we do in the ED?

- **Neurologic exam**. These bedside "brain tests" include asking you to do certain movements, such as raising your eyebrows, puffing out your cheeks, tracking a moving object, and balance testing.
- **CT scan**. This imaging test can rule out serious problems such as bleeding in or around the brain. It is not necessary for everyone, as there are downsides to every test. (See textbox on page 15, "Common Investigations Explained" for what this test involves.)

For more signs and symptoms of concussion, and a helpful guide on how to return to activity, visit Parachute Canada's website (Parachute.ca). This is a national charity dedicated to injury prevention.

Eczema

This is a troubling condition that causes long-term itchy, red, slightly scaly skin.

- **Try not to scratch.** Scratching causes more itching and swelling, leading to an itch-scratch vicious cycle. Instead, try cooling measures such as ice or a cool gel pack.
- **Avoid hot baths or showers.** These can trigger an itch.
- **Lock in moisture to prevent dryness**. After a bath or shower, apply an *emollient* to the skin right away. I find the majority of moisturizer lotions to be too thin and watery, so they don't last. I suggest mixing a plain, hypo-allergenic, fragrance-free lotion with a thicker ointment such as Vaseline (petroleum jelly). The result is an oily cream that still spreads easily over just-wet skin, but has staying power. Sometimes repeating this "shower and slather" twice a day helps my skin.
- **Consider dilute bleach baths**. This is a trick that has been better studied in kids but can be used in adults as well. The idea is to reduce the bacteria count on the skin (don't worry, we all have bacteria on our skin!) that can contribute to itching and inflammation when eczema is bad. How? Add about a cup of regular household bleach or less to a bathtub at least half-full of lukewarm water and mix well. The smell should be similar to a regular public swimming pool. Soak for 10 to 15 minutes. You can rinse off afterwards to avoid bleaching towels and bath mats.

Fainting

Fainting is a common condition that causes some people to worry enough to come to the ED. Most of the time it is not from a serious cause, especially if the person is young and otherwise healthy. Speak to a doctor or nurse if you are concerned.

Typically, a person will get a "warning" lasting seconds to minutes. This could be a combination of any of the following:

- Light-headedness
- Flushing, heat sensation, or sweats

- Nausea
- Blurry or "tunnel" vision
- Muffled sounds

And a regular fainting episode causes a brief loss of consciousness, less than a minute approximately. Witnesses might notice:

- Brief unresponsiveness and/or confusion
- Some occasional muscle twitching or jerks of arms or legs
- Regular but slowed breathing
- A possible repeat event if the person tries to sit or stand too quickly after waking

There are several things that can trigger these episodes including:

- Prolonged sitting or standing
- Standing up too quickly
- A hot environment
- A painful event (such as a needle poke)
- Recent illness, dehydration, or significant alcohol intake
- Missed meals or sleep
- Having just urinated or passed a bowel movement

We think the number one cause of fainting is *vasovagal*, which causes a relatively lower amount of blood or blood pressure getting to the brain. The vagus nerve is the anti-adrenaline nerve, which "turns down the volume" on your heart rate and blood pressure. Your brain tries to restore blood flow to your heart and brain by getting your body horizontal any way it can. So, a person who has just fainted should stay laying down for a while until all the symptoms clearly pass before slowly trying to sit, and eventually stand.

In these classic descriptions above, the chance of us finding anything wrong in the ED is very low. Tests that may be done, other than checking vital signs, include an ECG, blood sugar reading, and pregnancy test if applicable. Most people end up going home without any definite cause found.

Here are some fainting red flags that should prompt a person to come to the ED to get checked out:

- An older person or someone with chronic medical problems.

- Multiple home medications or recent changes.
- Severe pain associated (head, neck, chest, back, belly, or from an impact injury).
- Fainting during exercise.
- Tongue biting, incontinence, or severe and prolonged shaking to suggest seizure (which tends to be followed by a much longer period of unresponsive drowsiness lasting minutes).
- Losing consciousness without any warning at all
- Family history of sudden death in childhood or young adulthood. This could be a clue to rare heart structure or rhythm problems that can be inherited.

If You're Prone to Fainting, Can You Prevent an Episode When You Get a Warning?

YES!

First, try to get your head lower to the ground by sitting (even with your head towards your knees), squatting, or laying down if you can do so easily without standing and walking far. It's often when people try to get up, or wait too long and "push through" that they then faint.

Next are **counter-pressure techniques** you can do to reduce your chances of passing out. They involve **isometric exercises** to tighten muscles that might help pump more blood volume up to your brain.

Try any or all of these maneuvers:

- **Grip your hands** into tight fists several times, holding them tight for as long as you can.

- **Grip your hands** tight together next to your belly-button, using your arms to try to pull them apart to the sides of your body.

- **Heel raises** – from sitting or standing, push your toes firmly into the ground and raise your heels up to clench your calf muscles.

- **Buttock clenching** – tighten the muscles as long as you can, then release and repeat.

See also:

https://my.clevelandclinic.org/health/articles/counter-pressure-techniques

Gastroenteritis, a.k.a. "Stomach Flu"

Many people go to the doctor when they or their children have bouts of vomiting and diarrhea. They might also have fever and chills. After multiple bowel movements, there might even be a small amount of bright red blood on wiping or in the toilet bowl. Often the cause is either an infection, like a virus, or from something they ate. Multiple people in the household may have some symptoms around the same time, especially if it's from an infection. To prevent spread, it's very important for everyone to wash their hands well and frequently, especially before handling food or drinks.

Handwashing vs. Hand Sanitizer... Did You Know?

This is one scenario where even hand sanitizer is not as good as good old soap and water. Hand sanitizer *does not* kill some of the microbes that cause infectious diarrhea, such as Norovirus or Clostridium difficile!

Much of the time, this condition can be treated at home initially:

- **Treat the nausea first**:

  Option 1) Dimenhydrinate (brand name: Gravol) (see Medicines Everyone Should Have at Home, **page 72**)

  If Gravol pills don't stay down, there are a few options you can try:

    - Children's chewable Gravol. Even adults can benefit from a dose of this formulation. One children's tablet can be chewed and swallowed, or crushed and placed under the tongue. [15]

- Suppositories for rectal administration provide another way of getting Gravol in.

Option 2) Inhaled rubbing alcohol (isopropyl alcohol)

- Smelling rubbing alcohol has been shown to be more effective than placebo in the ED. This method has also been studied for nausea after operations requiring anaesthetic.
- If you have the single-use alcohol-wipe squares like we use at the hospital, go ahead and sniff those. Otherwise, you can apply a capful of liquid to a face cloth, makeup remover pad, or cotton ball.
- *Do not drink* this liquid, as it can be harmful, and try not to get it in your eyes.

- **Treat the fever and chills** with acetaminophen or ibuprofen. Wait a little while for the nausea to settle before adding this step.
- **Stay hydrated and replace those electrolytes** (the essential minerals your body needs) that your body is losing.

  - The priority is to replenish the fluids and electrolytes. Getting calories from solid food is much less important in the first few days of illness.
  - Drink *small* amounts of liquid frequently but spaced apart. When your guts are sensitive, if you drink too much too quickly, it can trigger vomiting. In children, for example, I often send parents home with a syringe so they can give 5 mL (one teaspoon) of fluid into the kid's mouth every 5 minutes or so. In adults, use this same principle to sip small amounts regularly. Even if it seems like that fluid is running straight

---

15   Scavone, J. M. "Diphenhydramine kinetics following intravenous, oral, and sublingual dimenhydrinate administration." *Biopharm Drug Dispos, 11.* (1990): 185-189. doi:10.1002/bdd.2510110302.

through you when you head to the bathroom, some of it is getting absorbed.

- Drink more than just plain water. If you think of your sweat and how salty that is, it gives you some idea of what you're losing through vomit and diarrhea. You can easily buy packages of oral rehydration salts such as Gastrolyte, which you mix with water yourself, or pre-mixed solutions such as Pedialyte. There are even Pedialyte freezies that some kids enjoy more, and they are great because a child can't consume too much too quickly when they are frozen.

- Here are some other solutions with my comments:

GREAT	Oral rehydration salts (such as Gastrolyte)	Convenient and cost-effective, especially when you mix it yourself
	Oral rehydration pre-mixed solutions (such as Pedialyte)	Ready to use. Freezies are often enjoyed.
FAIR	Half-strength apple juice (half apple juice with half water).[16]	For mild and early symptoms
	Half-strength Gatorade (half Gatorade with half water)	
POOR	Homemade combinations of salt, sugar, and water.	Errors in mixing could cause harm if measurements are incorrect
	Plain water	No electrolytes. This can become a problem if the body's sodium and potassium levels get too low.

16   Freedman S. B. "Effect of dilute apple juice and preferred fluids vs. electrolyte mainte-nance solution on treatment failure among children with mild gastroenteritis: a random-ized clinical trial." *JAMA, 315*. (2016): 1966-74. doi: 10.1001/jama.2016.5352.

Cannabinoid Hyperemesis Syndrome (CHS)

A condition that we are seeing much more of since legalization of marijuana involves *cyclical vomiting*. One of the hallmarks is that people often feel better when they take a hot shower or bath during an episode.

Often CHS occurs in people who use cannabis daily, and it can be quite stubborn to treat with our mainstay anti-nausea medications. As a result, we need to use antipsychotic medications (like haloperidol) to treat the vomiting. There is also capsaicin cream, which is derived from hot-peppers, that can be applied to the stomach instead of using direct heat.

The only way to stop and prevent these episodes is to quit using marijuana long-term. It can take weeks to months of avoidance for the symptoms to finally disappear.

Sometimes it is hard to convince patients that marijuana is the likely culprit because:

- CHS is a relatively new condition that we are still learning about, and

- Some cancer patients *treat* nausea with medical marijuana, but they have a different underlying cause for nausea and vomiting.

- When people abstain from marijuana for only a short period of time there may be no improvement. The body may have stored some of the cannabinoids in areas such as fat-cells so it takes a lot longer to clear than chemicals that are just in your bloodstream.

There is no specific test we can do to prove that vomiting is from CHS. Talk to your doctor for more specific guidance. In the ED, we can help temporarily relieve symptoms for those with severe or prolonged vomiting.

Mild Burns

Thermal burns frequently occur when a hot liquid is accidentally splashed on an area of skin. That area of your body continues to get damaged until it cools down. To minimize the amount of healthy skin that gets affected, gently run the scalded area under cool tap water for ten to twenty minutes continuously.

Mild burns (that look and feel like a sunburn) can usually be treated with pain medication (such as ibuprofen) and by covering it with an ointment such as Polysporin. The oily nature of an ointment acts as a barrier from the surrounding air so there is less pain. Very light gauze can be placed on top of the ointment to prevent it from getting rubbed away. However, do not apply a thick or heavy dressing that can trap the heat in.

If treating a mild burn at home, watch for signs of infection that may appear a few days afterward: spreading redness, warmth, tenderness, and swelling to skin that was not affected before. This potentially needs antibiotic pills that a doctor would prescribe.

BEWARE:

- Blistering suggests a deeper burn.
- Lack of pain to an area of obvious burn injury is actually *bad,* as it may suggest damage to the deepest layers of the skin that include nerves that would sense pain.
- Sensitive areas are more likely to need medical attention (such as the face, hands, and genitals).
- Areas that bend and move (for example, over a joint) are also important to discuss with your doctor.
- Burns from electricity or chemicals.

Nasal Congestion

A lot of people seem very bothered by a congested ("stuffy") or runny nose. They may have a cold and feel like they can't breathe, or they have allergies and sneezing fits during the spring. Some people get a post-nasal (back of the nose) drip that can cause a cough. Other people develop ear pain and pressure and feel like they can't "pop" their ears. (This is because the inner ear drains via a tube to the back of the nose. The end of this tube is naturally sealed by your eardrum, so there's nowhere else for fluid and air to go and the pressure builds up. The same thing occurs with changes in altitude; you feel the pressure and your hearing changes.)

Luckily, we have inexpensive nasal sprays that work fast to solve these annoying symptoms. The one I recommend is xylometazoline (Brand name:

Otrivin). But from personal experience, it's hard to sniff up the right amount of medication when your nose is plugged. And squirting too much medication up there causes a bad taste and funny feeling at the back of your throat. I like to coach my patients on the following technique to get the medication to where you need it:

1) Blow one side of your nose to clear out as much gunk as you can.
2) Open the medication bottle and grab a piece of facial tissue. **Do NOT use toilet paper**, which dissolves too quickly. Good substitutes are makeup remover pads, cotton balls, or gauze.
3) Twist a corner of the tissue into a tight cone.

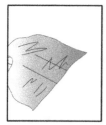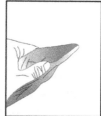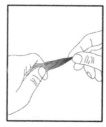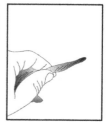

4) Apply a few drops of medication to the end of the tissue cone and place that medicated tip into your nose as far as you comfortably can.
5) Pinch and release the end of your nose a few times to get as much medication into contact with the inner surfaces of your nose.
6) Try breathing through your nose. If it hasn't improved, you can keep repeating these steps once or twice right away.
7) You may do the same process on the other side of your nose, if needed, with a fresh facial tissue.

If that doesn't work, another method is to:

1) Blow one side of your nose to clear out as much gunk as you can.
2) Lie down, tilt your head back, and squeeze several drops of medication into that nostril.
3) Pinch and release the end of your nose a few times to get as much medication into contact with the inner surfaces of your nose.
4) Repeat on the other side of your nose.

CAUTION: Do not use xylometazoline for more than five days before taking a few days off. Otherwise, if you use it for a long continuous period, there is a rebound effect where your symptoms will come back with a vengeance when you stop it.

Nosebleeds

Many people who come to the ED for a nosebleed have not tried a good technique for stopping it at home. Seeing your own blood can be distressing, but unless you are on a blood thinner, very rarely would you lose enough blood to need a blood transfusion. Using poor technique can actually make a nosebleed last longer.

Most nosebleeds come from the front part of your nose, along the wall (*septum*) separating your left from your right nostril. Fragile blood vessels in this area can leak after a violent sneeze or cough, with big changes in heat or humidity, or after picking your nose with a finger.

Here are some tips to stop your nosebleed more effectively:

DO:

- Pinch your nostrils together firmly in the soft front part just below where you can feel the harder bone.
- Tip your head forward.
- Sit down and rest quietly, which keeps your heart rate and blood pressure lower.
- Keep pressure firm and constant for at least 10 minutes.

DO NOT:

- Tip your head backwards. This position makes it more likely for blood to drip backwards to your throat and get swallowed.
- Frequently check or check too soon to see if your nosebleed has stopped. This disrupts the clot that your body is forming to stop the bleed.
- Necessarily use ice or an ice pack. It is unlikely that applying an ice pack to your neck or forehead will cause the blood vessels in your nostril to constrict. However, doing this probably won't hurt or help you.

When to go to the ED?

- If bleeding persists even after trying the above technique multiple times
- If the bleeding stays brisk and severe, coming out both nostrils at once
- If there is fainting and/or looking much paler than before

Talk to a nurse or doctor if you are unsure.

What can we do in the ED?

- We can insert a balloon or coated-gauze to apply pressure inside the nose to stop the bleeding. However, inserting it and leaving it in for a couple of days can be quite uncomfortable.
- Apply medications to the tissues of the inside of the nose to temporarily constrict (narrow) blood vessels.
- Possibly cauterize (destroy with heat) the leaking blood vessel causing the problem.

Skin Infections

Another reason people seek treatment is for skin infections. Any wound or break in the skin, even from a hair follicle, can cause a bacterial infection that can spread through the soft tissues in a condition we call *cellulitis*.

What are the signs of cellulitis?

- Redness, warmth, pain, and swelling that starts spreading from the initial area.
- Relatively slow spread over hours and even days.
- Sometimes, there can be a narrow red line that streaks up from this area towards your core. This is called *lymphangitis*.

Many times, this can be treated orally with antibiotics in pill form, prescribed by any doctor. Note that it can take 48-72 hours of treatment before the area of cellulitis starts shrinking.

You can help monitor the spread by either drawing a dotted line in pen around the borders of the redness and keeping track of the date, or take pictures from the same angle so you and your medical provider can watch for progression or improvement.

Sometimes the infection needs more urgent evaluation and treatment, and we want to see you in the ED, anytime of day or night. We want to make sure it's not a more serious problem like flesh-eating disease (*necrotizing fasciitis*), an abscess, or a bloodstream infection (*bactremia*).

BEWARE:

- Severe pain.
- Rapid spread over minutes to hours.
- Tenderness away from the area of redness, over normal-looking skin.
- The infection is around the eye.
- It hurts a lot to bend a joint.
- One central area is really firm or is draining pus
- Associated fever, chills, sweats, fainting, or just generally feeling unwell.

If you are worried, get assessed by a medical professional.

Is This Bite / Sting Infected?

When you are bitten or stung, say by a wasp, there is a toxin that causes a lot of inflammation to the surrounding skin. Sometimes it can look very dramatic, and similar to how a skin infection would look.

What helps me tell the difference is:

Itch versus Pain – I've noticed that envenomations are like allergic reactions and seem to cause some degree of itching as well as pain. Cellulitis, or a pure infection, is almost never itchy.

Timing – A one-time bite or sting is worst right away, or in the first 24 hours. An infection usually takes a while to ramp up, so it starts out small and tends to gradually get worse over days.

Previous History – If you've had previous exaggerated bite reactions to insects, it's likely to happen again.

Response to Medications – Treatment with ice packs, antihistamines, and topical steroids can make the redness and swelling of bites/stings better. However, they will not improve the skin when the cause is a bacterial infection.

Swallowing Stuff

Thankfully, many things that get swallowed pass through safely on their own. People come to the ED periodically when they or their children swallow something they didn't mean to. X-rays can be helpful to see where that foreign body is, but not everything shows up on an X-ray.

If you are worried, then you should come in for an assessment by a medical professional.

Be sure to come in for these higher-risk situations:

- There is a "stuck" feeling in the throat or chest. This can indicate that something is in the *esophagus* (or "swallowing-tube") and won't pass any further.
- The object is very long, wide, or sharp.
- The object is toxic (for example, laundry pods, batteries, household or workplace chemicals).
- The objects are magnetic (one might be safe, but two is definitely dangerous as they can trap your bowel in-between).
- There is abdominal pain or vomiting (which can signal bowel blockage).

Wounds and Wound Care

The way to stop bleeding from a wound is to put **firm direct pressure** on it.

Please don't use toilet paper! If you think about it, that paper product is designed to break up in water, unlike facial tissue which is made to stay together when wet. In the ED that becomes a big mess.

Bleeding from an Empty Tooth Socket

We often see patients who are bleeding from an empty tooth socket due to a recent dental extraction or a blow to the face that knocks out a tooth. The empty socket is small and a difficult area to get a finger or gauze into.

Here's a trick of the trade to keep in mind: **a teabag pressure dressing**

- Rinse a tea bag under warm tap water to soak the tea leaves inside.

- Squeeze the bag a few times to get rid of some of the concentrated tea.

- Next, rinse it under cold water (a colder compress may help blood vessels shrink closed).

- Squeeze out excess water

- Now the tea bag can be molded to fit into the tooth socket.

- Put firm pressure on the bag towards the area of bleeding for several minutes before releasing pressure. This can be done with a finger, or by biting down gently (which may be easier for areas in the back of the mouth).

Here are some often heard wound care myths that people (including some healthcare professionals) still believe.

MYTH # 1 – You need to clean your cut with _____ (fill in the blank with "peroxide" or "alcohol" or "iodine" or "sterile saline")

No! In fact, those first three solutions may even damage healthy tissue and cause worse wound healing.

There have been several studies that have compared irrigation of wounds with plain tap water versus sterile saline and there was no difference in the chance of infection between the two solutions.

The important thing is to clear out as much debris and microscopic bacteria as possible. The key is the volume of water, and sometimes the force. So, if it's not bleeding too profusely, just run it under the tap or shower nozzle for a few minutes. Make sure the water is cool or room temperature, not hot. Even water from a clean water bottle is fine.

MYTH # 2 – You need to get that cut fixed right away!

No. In the medical world, we used to think that fixing a cut within the first six hours was necessary, and some practitioners even avoided repair if it was "too late."

If the cut is bad, bleeding despite direct pressure, or you're worried about it, then come in to see a doctor, of course. If something's not working right, for example if your finger can't bend or straighten, then there could be a tendon injury and that can be harder to fix when it's delayed. In all of these cases, come to the ED.

If the cut is mild or moderate, then it's likely okay to wait till the morning when it's more convenient to get it assessed. You might be waiting a long time in the late evening, especially on the weekend, whereas if it's convenient to just come in the next morning, then you'll likely not have to wait as long to see the doctor.

MYTH # 3 – You can't bathe or shower after you get stitched up

Actually, you can bathe or shower right away after sutures or glue. You won't want to let it stay soaked or go in a public pool, but a wound that's been closed is quite water-tight. It's just good to keep it clean and relatively dry instead of letting it stay soaking wet.

If you've had glue to repair it, you've likely been told to avoid oil-based products such as Vaseline, conditioner, Polysporin, skin lotion, sunscreen, etc. That's because oils break down the glue (sooner than we'd like), but soap and water are fine.

MYTH # 4 – It's likely to get infected

Most wounds don't get infected, especially if you are healthy and the wound has been flushed out (see Myth # 1).

Some people (for example, smokers and diabetics) are more prone to infection. Wounds in some locations such as the shins and feet are more prone to infection. Certain types of wounds such as crush injuries or deep punctures are also more likely to get infected. If any of those apply to you, or it's a particularly dirty wound to begin with, some doctors will consider putting you on antibiotics to prevent infection, so consider getting it looked at. It's not always necessary—often you can just watch and wait and closely monitor for signs of infection, such as increasing pain, fever, or spreading redness and warmth.

MYTH # 5 – You've already had a tetanus shot so you don't need another one

If you've had the recommended childhood immunizations, that's fantastic, because tetanus is routinely part of that. However, if it's been more than

10 years since your last booster or 5 years if the wound is particularly dirty or tetanus-prone (see below), then you may need a tetanus shot even if you don't need the wound repaired. Some public health units or pharmacies can give you a tetanus shot, so if that is all you need you may be able to skip the emergency room if you can get immunized an alternate way.

Special precautions for a few types of wounds

The classic worry patients have is when they have "stepped on a rusty nail." What if I told you that I'm *less* worried about that situation, which tends *not* to cause infection as much as people fear, and *more concerned* about the following four types of wounds?

- Bites

    - Minor bites can be flushed under tap water.
    - Most bites will benefit from a few days of preventative antibiotics because the risk of infection is so high. This would include **cat and dog bites**, and wounds caused by **another person's** teeth (what we call a "fight bite").
    - Timing of these antibiotics is not consistently so urgent that an immediate visit to the ED is necessary. A walk-in clinic doctor should be able to sort it out, especially because bite wounds don't often need to be stitched closed.
    - The rare case of a possible **bat** bite does need a visit to the ED, however, because of the risk of rabies, a disease that is always fatal without treatment!

- Puncture through footwear

    - This doesn't seem to get enough public attention, but I think it's *really* important to know.
    - If you step on a nail with bare feet, it's usually not too much of a problem because the bacteria on the skin (*Staphylococcus and Streptococcus*, "staph and strep") are relatively easy to kill.
    - However, if a nail **punctures through a shoe, sneaker, or sandal**, the bacteria that grows there can be a big problem. It's called *Pseudomonas* and only a few antibiotics work well against it. Plus, it can even cause a bone infection

(*osteomyelitis*) that can be a big problem and need prolonged treatment.

- For those reasons, when the skin is punctured through footwear, seek medical attention. I generally recommend starting a
prescription for an antibiotic called ciprofloxacin, unless there
are reasons not to (such as allergy).

- Skin breakage in natural water

  - Cuts, bites, or punctures (from a fish hook, for example)
  that occur in lakes, rivers, and oceans may get infected with
  different bacteria (*Vibrio* and *Aeromonas*).

  - Be sure to mention that you were in **freshwater or saltwater**
  to your doctor if you are seeking help for the wound or
  possible infection.

  - You may then be prescribed more than one antibiotic to cover
  the additional organisms that you may have been exposed to.

- Tetanus-prone wounds

  - A dirty wound (e.g. contaminated with dirt, feces, soil
  or saliva)
  - A puncture wound
  - Wounds caused by a burn, frostbite, or crushing

For persons who have *not* had a full series of vaccinations before (which
includes three doses of tetanus vaccine), and any of the above characteris-
tics apply to the wound, then come to the ED. There is an *immune-globulin*
injection we give called TIG that can help mop up tetanus toxin for people
who did not previously complete their vaccinations.

Not So Common... But May Save You a Trip to the Emergency

I've chosen a couple of maneuvers that are as easy as party tricks to try for problems that sometimes bring people to the ED. I've chosen these because they are very safe, with few complications seen, or risks known. If you are unsure, or uncomfortable performing these on your own, you should come in.

Bruising Under a Fingernail or Toenail

If you accidentally hit your thumb with a hammer, or drop something heavy onto a toe, there is a painful condition that can develop. Basically, a bruise under the nail (*subungual hematoma*) forms, which can be especially painful because the growing blood pool is trapped under the nail.

When the new dark purple area is in the middle of the nail, treating this condition is easy to do and quickly relieves the pain. Basically, it involves making a small hole in the nail to allow that fluid to leave, reducing the pressure underneath.

In the ED, my favorite way to do this is to use a large-bore needle that I can spin by hand to drill through the nail surface. It doesn't hurt, and I stop after liquid comes out of the hole, and before the needle reaches any soft tissue underneath.

At home, a method that has been described involves a paperclip and a candle:

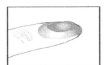 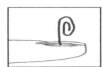 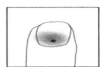

- Partially uncoil a paperclip so that there is a straight blunt metal end.
- Holding the remaining coil of paperclip like a handle, heat up the very tip of the metal for a few seconds.
- Avoiding the borders of the nail that have skin there, gently apply the hot tip to the nail overlying the dark purple region of bruising, being careful not to go too deep at first.
- If the hole has reached the fluid, then you should see a little fluid leaking out. At that point, you can stop. Squeeze the surrounding normal part of the nail to drain as much fluid as you can. When you're done, cover the hole with a bandage to sponge up anything further.
- If there is no fluid and no new pain, then you likely haven't gone far enough, so it is OK to repeat the heating of the paperclip tip and applying it to the hole you've started.

Nursemaid's Elbow *("pulled elbow" or radial head subluxation)*

In little kids who are able to walk on their own but need a helping hand at times, a parent or caregiver will often **pull** a child by **one** of their arms, say when crossing a street, getting off a bed, or out of a tub. If this motion causes an immediate and lasting pain in the elbow region, and the child no longer wants to bend their elbow, then this is almost certainly the diagnosis. What happens is one of the forearm bones (the radius) is slightly dislocated from the upper arm bone (the humerus) at the elbow joint. It is not a true dislocation like we see with shoulders, for example.

As long as the child is under 5 years old and the cause of pain is *not* from a fall or blow to the area (that may signify a break and need X-rays), it is safe to try the following quick treatment. It is, actually, very easy to accomplish. Called a *"reduction"* in medical terminology, it's one of the more satisfying procedures I do because it works so well, so quickly, and so dramatically. I have had astute triage nurses tell me a child has come in with this condition, and I can have the child fixed before they're even done registering the paperwork!

Here's how to try this at home:

- Prepare yourself for the child to be a bit anxious and reluctant.
- Think of the "Queen's Wave," and how she rotates her wrist and forearm. Or practice opening and closing an imaginary doorknob as

far as you can in each direction with your own hand. This is one of the two movements necessary to return the child's arm back to normal.

- Next think of lifting a dumbbell in a biceps curl. Bending the arm in this way until the hand nearly touches the shoulder on the same side is the second movement involved.
- Combining these two movements will be the route to success!
- Now use one hand to hold the child's elbow that they are not moving. You will know the procedure is done when you feel a little "click" in the elbow with your hand.
- With your other hand, take the child's hand and 1) bend the elbow like a full biceps/dumbbell curl while simultaneously 2) turning the child's wrist like in the doorknob opening fully.
- If you do not feel a "click" similar to when you "crack your knuckles," then try bending the elbow fully again with the wrist turning the doorknob closed fully.
- The child will not typically resist you, so it will be possible to rotate fully in each direction.

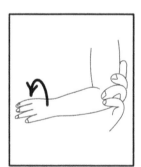 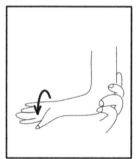 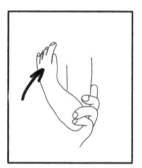

To know if you are successful, just wait a few minutes. When the child calms down and learns that their arm no longer hurts, they should begin using it again, as normal.

Voila!

If there is any leftover problem or pain with movement, then seek medical attention. Remember not to try this sequence if there was an actual fall or direct blow to the arm.

To prevent this from occurring, <u>avoid pulling a young child by only one arm</u>. Always hold onto both of their arms when lifting them up.

Something Up the Nose

One reason for parents to bring their child to the ED is because the child has stuck something somewhere. Some locations like the ear, eye, or nether regions (up the vagina or the "bum") require specialized equipment and careful medical attention. However, there is one instance where the parent can try something safely and easily at home. The location is the nose, as when little kids put a pea or a bead up their nose. I actually get the caregiver to first try this trick in the ED with a bit of coaching before I try to grab the item. This trick will work better for an object that doesn't have a hole through it, like a pea rather than a bead.

Here's how to try "The Mother's Kiss" technique, so named because it is often the mom who brings the child in:

- Tell the child you're going to kiss them on the lips to get the object out.
- Have some tissue ready in case you are successful.
- Get the child lying down on their back (such as on the couch or their bed) or sitting in a chair with their head supported.
- Next, using one finger, block the nostril that *doesn't* have the object in it.
- Ask the child to open their mouth a tiny bit. Or, pull the child's chin down with your other hand so their lips are parted.
- Go in for a kiss and form a seal around their mouth.
- Finally, give a forceful sharp puff of air by blowing as if you were trying to blow out a distant candle.
- If you have a good mouth seal and their other nostril is blocked, there's nowhere else for the air to go than out the nostril with the foreign object in it, and with luck, it will be blown out.
- Try this a few times. If nothing comes shooting out, then do seek medical attention.

Vertigo *(benign paroxysmal positional vertigo, BPPV)*

Vertigo is one of the most common causes of quick onset spinning sensation in healthy adults. It mainly begins suddenly, for example when you wake up or having just bent forward, and often includes intense nausea and vomiting. Turning rapidly makes it worse, whereas staying very still makes it temporarily go away. If it doesn't come and go, but is constant and causes you to be unable to sit or stand upright easily, it is *not* BPPV and you should go to your nearest ED.

Vertigo is caused by "ear rocks" (tiny crystals called *otoliths*) in the inner ear, specifically, in the fluid-filled semicircular canals. When these little crystals are dislodged, they disturb your body's ability to sense movement and head position, and this causes you to feel very nauseous.

If you have significant nausea, consider taking an over-the-counter medication to reduce it (see Medicines Everyone Should Have at Home, page 72). Then, you can try certain exercises to move these crystals into a better position so that vertigo troubles you less and less. **These exercises are known as Epley's Maneuver.**

You can find the sequence of exercises online in picture and video format (see my website DrVoon.com for links). From an initial sitting position, you slowly go through a series of motions that lets gravity shift the otoliths. If you do indeed have BBPV, moving through each step will cause some motion sickness and nausea. Typically, the spinning will be delayed by a few seconds and lasts less than a minute, before settling down when you're perfectly still. Wait for 30 to 60 seconds between steps to allow the otoliths to drift to where you are repositioning them.

- Step 1 – Sitting up in bed, looking straight ahead. This is the starting position.
- Step 2 – Lay back slowly until you are on your back, with your head turned to one side, as if you were shoulder-checking. It doesn't matter which side you start with. We'll repeat the cycle, eventually, on the other side.
- Step 3 – Without turning your head back to neutral, roll on to your side, in the same direction as your head is turned.

- Step 4 – Continue to turn your head as far as you comfortably can, so that you are now looking towards the ground.
- Repeat Steps 1-4. The second time you try this, you can try turning the opposite way (left or right). If one side is noticeably worse than the other, this is the direction you should keep repeating. The more you do these exercises, the better your positional vertigo should be.

Other tips:

- To make the Epley Maneuver more effective, you can place a pillow behind you, closer to your body than you would normally place it for sleep. The pillow should be in the area of your shoulders and neck when you are laying on your back, so that your head is tilted back a little bit. In the ED, we have stretchers that we can tilt so that your feet are a little bit higher than your head to do the same thing.
- Call your local physiotherapist. Some are specially trained in *vestibular rehabilitation* and can help guide you through these movements during an appointment.
- Sleep in a recliner at night for a while, or with your head and torso propped up on several pillows. This can help prevent the ear rocks from getting disturbed again.

APPENDICES

Appendix 1. ABCs of Prevention

Every day in the ED, we see countless patients whose injuries or illness could have been lessened by taking simple precautions or acting quickly. Of course, not all emergency visits are preventable, but as the old saying goes, "An ounce of prevention is worth a pound of cure."

A is for Aspirin – If you or someone else is having the signs of a heart attack, call 9-1-1 and chew two 81-mg tablets of aspirin. Do not treat suspected strokes with aspirin.

B is for Boating and water safety – Be respectful of the water; drownings happen quickly and quietly. Follow all boating safety rules. Wear your personal flotation device (PFD, "lifejacket"). Be vigilant when children are near water, no matter how shallow. Swimming lessons are important for kids and adults.

C is for CPR – Even "Compression-Only CPR" from a bystander increases the chances of survival for a person with a cardiac arrest. [17]

Compared to standard CPR with rescue breaths, "Hands-Only" CPR is simpler. In addition, a witness is more likely to volunteer to start CPR before a paramedic arrives. While formal training is recommended, pushing on the chest to keep blood pumping is still more effective than doing nothing. Good Samaritan laws protect you from problems that may arise after helping in a life-threatening emergency. The basic method is to:

- "Push fast and deep" by

    - Compressing down on the front of the chest, enough to flatten it by about a third
    - Then releasing fully to allow the chest to bounce back to normal
    - Repeating the steps above twice per second

---

17   American Heart Association. "Compression-only CPR increases survival of out-of-hospital cardiac arrest." ScienceDaily, 1 April 2019. www.sciencedaily.com/releases/2019/04/190401075158.htm (accessed August 22, 2020).

D is for Diet – A healthy diet is an essential part of overall good health and plays an important role in preventing chronic illnesses. Chances of getting acute painful conditions such as gout or kidney stones can be reduced with dietary changes. Special diets are important for those with diabetes or poor kidney function.

E is for Eye protection – Eye safety goggles prevent sports injuries (for example getting a squash ball in the eye), chemical injuries, and accidental injuries when working with power tools. We see many people for foreign bodies in the eye because they were not wearing proper eye-shielding protection.

F is for Flu shot – The annual flu shot is your best defense against influenza, which sadly kills thousands of Canadians every year. I get mine every year, and so does every emerg doc that I know.

G is for Gauze – In your home first-aid kit, have a supply of clean gauze in case you need to need to wrap a heavily bleeding cut until you can get to the ED. Four-inch squares are quite versatile. I would suggest stocking those plus some gauze rolls to wrap around an extremity.

H is for Helmets – The best protection against concussions and traumatic brain injuries that occur during sports is a helmet. Wear the helmet designed for the sport. Make sure it fits properly and do it up! If riding a motorized vehicle, choose a helmet with more protection than just a skull cap.

I is for Internet – Use it wisely! Visit reputable sites to learn more about your health, but please leave the diagnosing to real doctors versus "Dr. Google"! I have provided a list of links and resources on my site DrVoon.com.

J is for "Just a little bit at a time" – There has been an increase in the number of people showing up in the ED for unwanted effects of marijuana. The potency of marijuana has gone up considerably from decades ago. Edibles are especially problematic because of large variability in THC content. The effects are slow to start, making it easy to take too much at the beginning, and they last extra long, causing people to stay anxious, paranoid, or uncoordinated for a number of hours.

K is for Knowledge – Be involved in your healthcare. Ask questions, and ask to have key answers written down! Be sure you understand the information you get from your healthcare team.

L is for Listen to guided meditations – There is good evidence that mindfulness training and practice are helpful for a wide range of conditions: anxiety, depression, chronic pain, addiction relapse prevention, insomnia, eating healthier, and more. There are studies showing positive effects for students, athletes, healthcare workers, teachers, business people, police and military, and even lawyers! It's probably something that everyone can benefit from.

M is for Moles – New moles or changes to an existing mole can be a sign of skin cancer. See your family doctor if you notice these changes. Look up the "ABCDE's of Melanoma" for red flags and example images.

N is for Naloxone kit – This kit is available free from numerous pharmacies and can save the life of a person who has overdosed on opioids such as street fentanyl, or if you have prescription opioids in the house.

O is for Overdose prevention – Make sure medications are out of reach of children, and ensure that alcohol and cannabis products are not in places that can be easily accessed by children. Read the instructions on labels before taking or combining any medications. People using recreational substances should never do so alone.

P is for Poison control – Have the phone number for your local Poison Control centre in your cell phone and written beside your landline. They can provide advice over the phone, including telling you whether you should go to the ED.

Q is for Quit smoking – No matter how long you have been smoking, your health risks are reduced if you can cut down or quit. We see many people with breathing difficulties from COPD (chronic obstructive pulmonary disease) as a result of years of smoking. Wounds heal slower in smokers. Heart attacks and strokes are more likely if you smoke.

R is for Road safety – Always wear your seatbelt. Don't text and drive! We like to think we can multitask, but in reality we just shift attention quickly—and not fast enough to prevent serious crashes when operating a vehicle. Obey speed limits. Talk to elderly and medically at-risk family members about testing fitness to drive safely (https://www.driveable.com). Take a training course if you plan to ride a motorcycle. Pedestrians, make sure you are *very* visible at night.

S is for Sun protection – Protect yourself from short-term problems like sunburn, heatstroke, and heat exhaustion, and from the long-term negative effects of the sun, such as skin cancer.

T is for Teeth – Poor dental health has been shown to be related to an assortment of chronic health problems. Take good care of your teeth and gums and visit your dentist regularly.

U is for Understanding your medications – Talk to your pharmacist and family doctor about your medications, especially if you are unsure what they do or if you are interested in stopping them. De-prescribing is the term for reducing or stopping medications that may no longer be beneficial or that risk causing harm if taken too long. Sometimes our bodies change to the point where the dose of medication we needed before becomes too strong for our current needs. This can lead to falls, fainting, electrolyte abnormalities, and delirium. See https://www.deprescribingnetwork.ca/ for more information.

V is for Vaccines – Children need all their immunizations, but older adults need vaccines too. Check with your family doctor to see if you are eligible to receive the shingles vaccine and the vaccine that prevents bacterial pneumonia. Also, before you travel make sure you get all the recommended vaccines for the area you are visiting. Tetanus booster shots are needed every 10 years.

W is for Water – Prevent dehydration when out in the sun or playing sports by drinking enough water. Also, know that it is possible to become "water toxic" (*hyponatremic*)—diluting your body's electrolytes by drinking *too much* plain water without replacing the salts as well.

X is for eXtra medication – There are certain medications you want to be sure you always have enough of:

Puffers for asthma

Epinephrine for anaphylaxis

Psychiatric medications (because missing doses can sometimes cause people to feel quite unwell)

Diuretics or "water pills" for congestive heart failure

Blood thinners for clots and atrial fibrillation.

Some provinces allow pharmacists to renew medications without a doctor's note if you are unable to get a hold of your doctor or visit the nearest clinic.

Y is for Youth, mental health, and substance use – In Canadian youth, cannabis-related hospitalizations are more common than hospitalizations for any other known substance, followed by hospitalizations related to alcohol.[18] I am concerned about the risks of THC on the growing brain, especially that psychosis can be triggered, and it is sometimes irreversible.

Z is for Zinc oxide – This cream is ideal for preventing and treating diaper rash, as well as other skin problems where moisture is a factor, such as *candida* (skin fold "yeast infections"). I find mixing it with petrolatum (Vaseline) makes it easier to spread.

---

18   Canadian Institute for Health Information. "Hospital Stays for Harm Caused by Substance Use Among Youth Age 10 to 24, September 2019." Ottawa, ON: CIHI; 2019. https://www.cihi.ca/sites/default/files/document/hsu-youth-report-2019-en-web.pdf.

Appendix 2. Internet Sites I Trust

It can be difficult to find reliable health information on the Internet. Some sites are excellent and many are not. Many of the sites I refer my patients to upon discharge from the ED don't show up on the first few pages of popular search engines so I've compiled several below. Updated links can also be found on my website DrVoon.com.

I cannot attest to the accuracy of all the advice the following sites contain. Although, from what I have seen, they are excellent resources with information targeting the general population in a clear and concise way.

These are just some of the sites with broad applicability that I refer people to every shift. Each physician will often know their local resources, with websites specific to your home area you can be pointed to. That is why it can be vital to form a good relationship with a doctor in your own community that can see you on an ongoing basis.

Readers should not rely on Internet sites as a substitute for talking to a doctor.

Anxietycanada.com

I refer patients to this website every single day. It is amazing how prevalent stress and anxiety are and how they affect our well-being. Everyone could benefit from much of the information here and there are helpful topics addressing everything from sleep to worry, facing fears, and managing obsessions.

The site offers a scientifically-based free app called **Mindshift CBT** to download.

For anxiety in children and youth, there are dedicated sections for each, along with videos and quick tips.

Choosing Wisely

www.choosingwisely.org

As they describe themselves, "the mission of Choosing Wisely is to promote conversations between clinicians and patients by helping patients choose care that is:

- Supported by evidence
- Not duplicative of other tests or procedures already received
- Free from harm
- Truly necessary"

Their aim is "to help patients and their providers get on the same page by targeting tests and procedures of questionable benefit, yet still commonly performed. Avoiding unnecessary care can help reduce the risk of iatrogenic (caused by the physician and health care system) complications and unwanted side effects."

Familydoctor.org

- From the Academy of Family Physicians in the USA
- Great illustrations and easy to read
- Many conditions covered
- Some of the diagnostics and therapeutics mentioned are a bit different from Canadian and European practice patterns

greatergood.berkeley.edu

The Greater Good Science Centre (GGSC) is a site I've discovered and have been sharing with my physician colleagues to improve their wellness. It is relevant, however, to everyone.

A non-profit organization, the GGSC offers excellent evidence-based suggestions in many formats including videos, podcasts, articles, an email subscription, and happiness calendars. There is an entire section on the Keys to Well-Being that draws on results of studies that look at human happiness.

Mental health is a huge component of what we see in the ED and in family medicine offices around the globe.

HealthLinkBC.ca

A lot of work has obviously gone into providing fact sheets on a large number of conditions that are searchable, easy to understand, and available in multiple languages. Look for the "Files List" on the website and you can browse alphabetically and sign up for email updates.

patient.info

From the UK, an award-winning and visually attractive website. It discusses many health conditions categorized into sensible groups. A unique feature is their "symptom-checker" that allows you to enter the region of the world you are in, your age, gender, and symptoms you might be experiencing. You will be given a list of common conditions to consider as well as rare, but worrisome, ones to not miss!

Johns Hopkins Medicine

https://www.hopkinsmedicine.org/health

- Health topics including various conditions and diseases; treatments, tests and therapies; wellness, prevention, and caregiving

National Organizations

Many national organizations have websites with reliable information, such as:

- Canadian Pediatric Society (CPS) https://www.caringforkids.cps.ca/
- Society of Obstetricians and Gynaecologists of Canada (SOGC) https://sogc.org/en/public-resources/en/content/public-resources/public-resources.aspx

Larger or Specialized Hospitals

Many hospitals offer trusted medical information on a wide variety of topics, for example:

- BC Children's Hospital (http://www.bcchildrens.ca/health-info/coping-support)
- Children's Hospital of Eastern Ontario (CHEO) (https://www.cheo.on.ca/en/resources-and-support/library-catalogue.aspx)
- Toronto Sick Kids Hospital (https://www.aboutkidshealth.ca/)

Provincial Health websites

Each province offers patient health information with local phone numbers to call. For example, Alberta offers a comprehensive website: https://myhealth.alberta.ca/health/Pages/default.aspx

A Google search for your province's ministry of health is a good place to start.

Appendix 3. Sample Medical History Summary

You can download and print this summary from my website DrVoon.com. Once you complete it, consider carrying it with you at all times in case of an emergency.

Full Name:

Date of birth:

Provincial health card number:

Private health insurance information (if applicable) (company, policy number, contact telephone number). Some medications and equipment are only covered with extended health benefits:

Home phone number:

Cell phone number:

Email:

Emergency contact / family (provide names, relationship to you and telephone numbers):

Family physician:

Names of other **treating specialists**:

Do Not Resuscitate order (attach signed and dated copy):

Active medical problems:

Prior medical problems:

Previous surgeries, **medical devices, or implants** (e.g. pacemaker, stent, hip replacement) (details and dates):

All **current medications** and any that you **recently stopped** (names and dosages):

- Prescribed:
- Over-the-counter:
- Any recently stopped or changed:

Allergies (include typical reaction and severity)

- Medication:
- Anesthetic:
- Other (e.g. foods, animals, insect stings):

Social History

- Smoker? If yes, how many packs a day, and for how many years? Have you quit?
- Alcohol? If yes, how many drinks a week? If you drink daily, when was your last drink?
- Cannabis?
- Other drugs?
- Living situation (for example, alone, married, supports, walker/cane)?
- Who can give me a ride home? What's their phone number?
- Is there a spare house key hidden or with a trusted person?

Appendix 4. Advance Directive

This is an important subject that we don't talk enough about as individuals, families, and societies.

If you have strong feelings about what actions related to your healthcare would be OK with you, and what would not be worth the risks, you can decide that *in advance*. *Directive* means that you are directing others as to what you wouldn't want to be done to you if you are in a health situation where you can't communicate that yourself. This is sometimes referred to as a "personal directive."

A "DNR" (Do Not Resuscitate order) is an example of an advance directive by a patient (who is mentally fit to do so at the time), essentially requesting, "If my heart were to stop or my lungs were to fail, do not perform CPR or attempt other heroics and invasive procedures."

What would you want to be done if something were to happen that caused your heart or lungs to stop, or if a catastrophic illness struck you? A stroke, a major brain bleed, an overwhelming infection? Everybody will have a different response and different reasons.

Nearly everyone who is younger, relatively healthy and active, with good mental function would choose to have every reasonable resuscitative effort attempted. However, you might choose differently if you had a chronic "non-fixable" condition, if your quality of life was deteriorating, or if you were in pain every day. As we get older, we have less ability to bounce back from a life-threatening illness or injury. The risk of only partial recovery also increases with the burden of illnesses you accumulate over your life. What I mean is that even if we were able to resuscitate you—restart your heart, breathe for you with a tube down your throat—there's a chance that your brain and other vital organs might have gone too long without blood flow and oxygen to fully recover.

How willing would you be to accept the risk of surviving in a weakened state, perhaps with some loss of function (of your arms, your legs, your ability to eat, your ability to think and remember)? Could you live with the possibility of complications from resuscitative efforts? Ribs break during CPR; kidneys fail and may require a lifetime of dialysis treatments.

This is the dilemma many people face at some point in time. I bring up this difficult subject because it can be extremely difficult to try to figure this out in the heat of the moment, for patients and their families, as well as their healthcare providers. Those who end up in the ED having already given it some thought, discussion, or even written those decisions down often have a smoother course with less distress.

Once you feel more informed, I recommend having a more personalized discussion with your Family Doctor. It is not an "all or nothing" choice, either. There are nuances where some interventions may be practical and others may not be.

Here are some websites you might find helpful while thinking about the subject more.

Dying With Dignity Canada

www.dyingwithdignity.ca

A national human-rights charity committed to improving the quality of dying, protecting end-of-life rights, and helping Canadians avoid unwanted suffering.

Their website offers province-specific planning kits and educational resources, including written material and webinars.

Healthlink BC

https://www.healthlinkbc.ca/health-feature/advance-care-planning

Information is available in multiple languages, including Chinese, Farsi, French, Korean, Punjabi, Spanish, and Vietnamese.

It's OK to Die when you are prepared

https://www.oktodie.com/

Dr. Monica Williams-Murphy is an American Emergency Medicine Physician and offers helpful advice in her book, blog, and website. You will find resources, a newsletter, and checklists.

MAID – Medical Assistance in Dying

In 2016, the Parliament of Canada passed federal legislation that allows eligible Canadian adults to request medical assistance in dying.

https://www.canada.ca/en/health-canada/services/medical-assistance-dying.html

Appendix 5. What Changes During a Pandemic?

The medical community knew a pandemic was coming. We just didn't know when or what it would look like. I remember sitting in a classroom before the turn of the millennium and learning that:

- Viruses have been around a lot longer than we have.
- Viruses can infect different animal species and sometimes jump from one type of host to another (like avian flu or swine flu starting in animal reservoirs and then evolving to infect humans).
- Some viruses mutate frequently—others develop and accumulate changes slowly over time.
- Some mutations make the virus weaker, but these mutations don't become predominant because they fail to spread as rapidly. When other random mutations make the virus more likely to evade our immune system, or transmit differently, these strains become head-line news.
- An epidemic, or widespread infectious disease, that spreads rapidly and globally is called a pandemic.

Humanity has had several "dress rehearsals" for SARS-CoV-2, the virus that causes COVID-19. The first SARS outbreak in 2003, for example, was something new that we were fortunate enough to contain.

At the time of publication, we are still trying to immunize and prevent the spread of the COVID-19 pandemic and we are uncertain what the future will hold. In some ways, it is a race between who can evolve faster: this strain of coronavirus, or the human species.

What has stayed the same?

We already know that some diseases are highly infectious, transmitting through the air or by droplets. For example, healthcare workers are always on the lookout for possible measles, tuberculosis, and chickenpox. Other diseases we see in the ED are spread by direct contact (touching) including infectious diarrhea, scabies, and MRSA (methicillin-resistant staphylococcus aureus).

We already isolate certain patients with infectious diseases as well as those with compromised immune systems. Gloves and hand hygiene have been a priority for decades.

Swabs for respiratory illness were already happening regularly for patients suspected to have the flu or whooping cough.

Emergency Departments are used to adapting

ED staff already have some pre-existing knowledge and training for contaminated patients, mass casualty incidents, and industrial accidents such as:

- Chemical—including pesticides, chlorine gas, tear-gas, or pepper-spray
- Biological—including anthrax, Ebola, and Norwalk norovirus
- Radiological and nuclear—including radioactive materials

I believe principles learned from these scenarios can be adapted early in a public health crisis, even if they derive from a new cause, to prevent spread to staff and other patients. Healthcare workers that gravitate towards Emergency Medicine tend to be quick to adapt, make use of what's available, and can make challenging situations work even when limited information is available.

How is the Emergency Department different now?

Arriving to the ED might look different during a pandemic. Some hospitals will have pre-screening by a greeter or ambassador. Staff in other departments may be using the phone to limit time spent in close proximity to patients.

Basic procedures like hand cleansing and mask-wearing are now practiced more diligently by staff. Now, hospitals are asking people entering to also perform these simple infection-control procedures. Unfortunately, there may be severe limitations on the number of people the ED can accommodate, so having family and visitors could be restricted.

Staff efforts at prevention also occur behind the scenes. Healthcare workers pre-pandemic used to show up to work sick, with a "tough it out" mentality. To avoid getting the virus ourselves and spreading it to others, we are now required to stay home. We may be wearing gloves and barrier layers more regularly—which can slow us down and make it harder for you to know who is who.

Locally, we saw a drop in the number of people arriving at the Emergency Department initially but that was short-lived. There may have been fewer car collisions but people still had strokes and heart attacks. Now, with many community doctors restricted to seeing patients virtually using telehealth, there may be fewer alternatives for patients to access care that requires a physical examination. Sadly, the mental health burden of a drawn-out pandemic has also taken a toll and we are seeing many people that have reached a crisis point.

What can you do?

When the public does their part, it helps us care for you. A strong public health response can help the health care system from getting overwhelmed. Become informed but understand that it is staggeringly easier to spread misinformation or disinformation than it is to correct it.

Appendix 6. Glossary

A&E – A term used in the UK and countries that mirror their healthcare model; it stands for "Accident & Emergency" …not the Arts & Entertainment channel.

Ambulatory – a person who is, on the whole, able to move themselves from one location to another. May also refer to a section of the Emergency for the "walking wounded."

Bed – A location in the ED or hospital; e.g. "Bed 8." Sometimes a stretcher in a room, or between curtain-like partitions, but maybe in an overflow area such as a hallway, or in front of a nursing station.

Chief Complaint – The primary reason why a patient has sought medical attention.

Code – Usually refers to a "Code Blue," which is a cardiac or respiratory arrest. There are other Code colors, which may vary by hospital, that alert staff to major issues.

CT Scan – "Computed Tomography" a.k.a. "CAT Scan." A patient is placed on a sliding platform that moves briefly through a doughnut-shaped machine that spins an X-ray generator and sensors to get a 3D view of internal organs and structures. The tube is not as deep as an MRI machine where a patient goes into a long tunnel. Claustrophobia is less of an issue than for an MRI for that reason, and because the scans take much less time.

DNR – Do Not Resuscitate. A directive given in advance by a patient (who is mentally fit to do so at the time) essentially requesting "If my heart were to stop or my lungs were to fail, do not perform CPR or attempt other heroics and invasive procedures." There can be varying degrees of intervention and different abbreviations to describe them.

ECG – Electrocardiogram, a.k.a. EKG (from the German origin *"Elektrokardiographie"*). This quick, simple, cheap, and non-invasive test gives us a snapshot of your heart and how it is beating. Stickers are applied to your chest and limbs and the electrical signals are recorded and printed out. It can signal if you are having or have ever had a heart attack. But it can also give clues about your electrolytes, show arrhythmias, warn us not to use certain medications, or hint at other life-threatening conditions. See also Holter Monitor.

ED – Emergency Department. This term is favored over Emergency Room (ER) because it better reflects the size and complexity of the system in which we work.

ERP – ER Physician (pronounced "urrp"), "Emerg Doc." I suppose EDP or EP don't have the same ring to them! In different places, we go by "Attending," as in Attending Physician, or a variety of other nicknames such as "Duty Doc," "Staff Doc," or "CO" for Casualty Officer.

FP or GP – Family Practitioners are doctors that specialize in Family Medicine and are experts in diagnosing and treating the whole person. With time and the relationship that grows as they get to know you better, they can take into account important factors in your life including your job, values, family, financial situation, previous trauma or addictions, and culture. A trusted Family Doctor can see you in the context of your life, help prevent problems, and screen for disease when appropriate. The term "General Practitioner" is leftover from a time when physicians could work as a primary care provider without additional training or certification in community healthcare. Now Family Practitioners have training, supervision, and experience in the difficult task of being a generalist.

Holter Monitor – A monitoring device like an ECG or portable cardiac monitor that a patient wears for a 24 to 48-hour period of time to try to "catch" any heart rhythm disturbances. May be combined with an event monitor where a person tracks when they have symptoms that might be related to the arrhythmia the doctor is tracking.

Inpatient – Once a physician decides to admit a patient to stay in the hospital, that person becomes an inpatient.

IV – Intravenous. Medications and fluids can be delivered straight into the bloodstream for faster therapeutic onset. A plastic tube sits on top of a sterile needle; both are inserted, but the needle comes out and only the plastic tube remains. There are numbers to indicate how big the diameter of the tube is, and how long the needle is.

LOS – Length of Stay. This is tracked on our computer system from the minute you register, and is one factor that helps us determine who needs to be seen next.

MAID – Medical Assistance in Dying. In 2016, the Parliament of Canada passed federal legislation that allows eligible Canadian adults to request medical assistance in dying.

https://www.canada.ca/en/health-canada/services/medical-assistance-dying.html

MRI – Magnetic Resonance Imaging. The benefit of this test is that no radiation is used. Finer detail can usually be achieved, different from what a CT scan (see above) can show. However, it can be slower, less accessible, louder, and more claustrophobia-inducing than other tests. Some things, such as bone and blood, maybe seen less well than on CT.

Outpatient – Emergency patients before they are given a "disposition plan" are outpatients. Also refers to patients sent home to await further testing or procedures upon call-back at a specific date or time.

Procedural Sedation – Some procedures are painful enough, yet necessary, that the doctor will offer medication so the patient doesn't feel or remember the event. Depending on the doctor's experience and the setting, they may be able to use an intravenous medication that only takes minutes to work, and wears off very quickly.

Resident – A doctor in name, having successfully completed medical school, they are still gaining experience "on the job." In order to practice independently, they must apply to and graduate from a two to five-year program of specialization, even if that specialization is Family Practice (which used to be known as GP or General Practice). They are paid a small amount and work semi-autonomously under the supervision of one or several experienced physicians. A senior resident may be responsible for teaching junior residents and medical students.

Sharps – Can include IV needles, sutures, and scalpels. They must be treated cautiously at all times by staff to prevent "occupational exposure" or "needlestick" injuries, which put providers at risk of acquiring an infectious disease, such as Hepatitis or HIV. Sharps must be disposed of diligently into special containers.

Splint – Unlike a cast, which fully encircles an injured body part, a splint helps stabilize an area like the wrist or ankle with *removable* protection so it moves less. There is usually a rigid side (fibreglass, plaster, or plastic) and a soft area to hold it on (gauze, wrap, or Velcro).

Stretcher – a.k.a. "gurney." A padded bed on wheels that allows a patient to be moved around on it. Assigned to one location (e.g. "Bed 6").

Trauma – Injury by force to a person's body, which can be further categorized as "blunt" (such as a vehicular collision) or "penetrating" (such as a knife-stabbing or gunshot wound).

Trauma Room – a.k.a. "Resuscitation Room" because it is not only for major trauma, but a designated location to handle the critically ill. It is kept stocked with life-saving equipment and medications, a cardiac monitor, defibrillator, oxygen, suction, and more. There is usually a lot of space surrounding one stretcher because many professionals act simultaneously on different parts of the body. Larger centres may, in addition, have one specifically for pediatric patients (children).

Ultrasound – This imaging test uses sound waves, like sonar in a submarine, instead of X-rays to look deep inside the body. In the ED, we use "bedside ultrasound" for a point-of-care "quick look" in certain cases. There is also a comprehensive version we call a "formal ultrasound," done by a technician and read by a radiologist. Ultrasound is safe for every patient, as there is no radiation involved.

Vital Signs – Heart rate (or pulse), breathing rate, blood pressure, and temperature. It can also include some key numbers such as level of consciousness, oxygen saturation, and blood sugar level.

Appendix 7. List of Side Bars

- This book is not for everyone! — Page XIV
- MYTH: If I call 9-1-1 and go to the ED by ambulance, I will be seen faster by a doctor. — Page 4
- Planning to Go? Plan to Come Back! — Page 6
- Electronic Health Records. — Page 9
- MYTH: "It doesn't look too busy…" — Page 10
- How to Put on a Hospital Gown. — Page 12
- What Do These Numbers and Lines on the Cardiac Monitor Mean? — Page 13
- Common Investigations Explained. — Page 15
- Scared of Needles? — Page 20
- What If You Don't Have a Family Doctor? — Page 22
- "Board to Tears" — Page 23
- Why See a Family Doctor? — Page 26
- Please Do Not Keep Asking the Nurses How Long It Will Be! — Page 33
- Patients or Patience? — Page 36
- How to Collect a Good Urine Sample. — Page 38
- Do Tell! — Page 39
- There's more to 8-1-1 Than a Nurse! — Page 41
- If You're Getting Really Anxious and Distressed While Waiting, What Can You Do? — Page 44
- Assume at Your Own Risk. — Page 53
- Medical Student Syndrome. — Page 59
- How to Tell if Someone May Be Having a Stroke. — Page 62
- Tips on Using Eye Drops. — Page 67
- When to Suspect Appendicitis. — Page 68
- MYTH: Don't take medications beforeyou see a doctor because it might "mask" the fever or pain. — Page 71
- Your Friendly Neighborhood Pharmacist. — Page 76
- Prevent Medication Overdoses! — Page 77
- Your Allergic Reaction Toolkit. — Page 85
- Choosing Wisely. — Page 86

- If You're Prone to Fainting, Can You Prevent an Episode When You Get a Warning?   Page 94
- Handwashing vs. Hand Sanitizer... Did You Know?   Page 95
- Cannabinoid Hyperemesis Syndrome (CHS).   Page 97
- Is This Bite / Sting Infected?   Page 103
- Bleeding from an Empty Tooth Socket.   Page 104

REFERENCES

Canadian Institute for Health Information. *NACRS Emergency Department Visits and Length of Stay by Province/Territory, 2018–2019.* Ottawa, ON: CIHI, 2019. Table 1, 6a, and 9.

Rui P., Kang K. *National Hospital Ambulatory Medical Care Survey: 2017 emergency department summary tables.* National Center for Health Statistics. https://www.cdc.gov/nchs/data/nhamcs/web_tables/2017_ed_web_tables-508.pdf.

Canadian Institute for Health Information. *NACRS Emergency Department (ED) Visits: Volumes and Median Length of Stay by Triage Level, Visit Disposition, and Main Problem, 2018–2019.*

"How to make the most of 811," CBC News, May 7, 2019, https://www.cbc.ca/news/canada/nova-scotia/how-to-make-the-most-of-the-811-service-1.5126002.

Harvard Health Publishing. *Drug Expiration Dates—Do They Mean Anything?* Last modified Dec. 13, 2019. *https://www.health.harvard.edu/staying-healthy/drug-expiration-dates-do-they-mean-anything.*

Browne E., "Expired Drugs in the Remote Environment," *Wilderness & Environmental Medicine* 30, 1 (2019): 28-34. https://doi.org/10.1016/j.wem.2018.11.003.

Oduwole O., Udoh E. E. "Honey for acute cough in children," *Cochrane Database of Systematic Reviews* (2018): Issue 4. DOI: 10.1002/14651858.CD007094.pub5.

Cohen P. A. "Emergency department visits and hospitalisations for adverse events related to dietary supplements are common," *BMJ Evidence-Based Medicine,* 21 (2016): 79.

Office of Dietary Supplements. "Evidence Based Review Program," National Institutes of Health. USA. Accessed July, 2020. https://ods.od.nih.gov/Research/Evidence-Based_Review_Program.aspx.

Geller, A. "Emergency Department Visits for Adverse Events Related to Dietary Supplements," *New England Journal of Medicine,* 373. (2015): 1531-1540. DOI: 10.1056/NEJMsa1504267.

Browne E., Peeters F., Priston M., Marquis P. T. Expired Drugs in the Remote Environment. *Wilderness Environ Med.* 2019;30(1):28-34. https://doi.org/10.1016/j.wem.2018.11.003.

Bad Science Watch. "NHP Marketing in Canada: A Survey of the Online Marketing of Natural Health Products for Cancer Treatment and Cure," Accessed July, 2020. https://badsciencewatch.ca/natural-health-product-retailers-sell-cancer-cures.

Scavone, J. M. "Diphenhydramine kinetics following intravenous, oral, and sublingual dimenhydrinate administration." Biopharm Drug Dispos, 11. (1990): 185-189. doi:10.1002/bdd.2510110302.

Freedman S. B. "Effect of dilute apple juice and preferred fluids vs electrolyte maintenance solution on treatment failure among children with mild gastroenteritis: a randomized clinical trial." *JAMA, 315.* (2016): 1966-74. doi: 10.1001/jama.2016.5352.

American Heart Association. "Compression-only CPR increases survival of out-of-hospital cardiac arrest." ScienceDaily, 1 April 2019. www.sciencedaily.com/releases/2019/04/190401075158.htm (accessed August 22, 2020).

Canadian Institute for Health Information. "Hospital Stays for Harm Caused by Substance Use Among Youth Age 10 to 24, September 2019." Ottawa, ON: CIHI; 2019. https://www.cihi.ca/sites/default/files/document/hsu-youth-report-2019-en-web.pdf.

I would like to thank my developmental editor Cynthia Lank, my illustrator Pauline Voon, and Carla Unger Photography for the head shot.

Many others helped make this book possible, whether they knew it or not, and it is with gratitude that I name a few of them.

ACKNOWLEDGMENTS

Raymond Aaron	Dermot Kelleher
Hugh Aitken	Ashley Kressner
Laureen Bali	Ken Lam
Tanya Bonell	Brian Lee
Keila Byron	Karen Lindsay
Dave Chilton	Trellia Loveless
Stewart Clark	James Heilman
Stephen Dalupan	Fraser MacKinnon
Olivia Dam	Andrew MacPherson
Jeffrey Eisen	Og Mandino
Kate Evans	Helen McColl
Cara Fitzgerald	Elizabeth McGrath
Rishi Gupta	Laura Monchak
Tristan Jones	Lindsay Monier-Williams

Christopher Morrow

May Mrochuk

Michelle Rico

Auna Ross

Peter Roberts, Q.C.

Jia Ting

Dianne Walter

Bruce Wright

Graeme Young

ABOUT THE AUTHOR

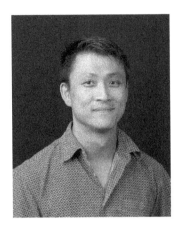

Dr. Frederick Voon is a Canadian Emergency physician who works in Victoria, B.C. He believes every patient would benefit from having information written down for them when they leave the hospital.

After graduating medical school in 2001, he completed residency training in Family Practice and Emergency Medicine. He has worked in clinic and hospital settings, both urban and rural, in British Columbia, Alberta, New Brunswick, Nova Scotia, and New Zealand.

Currently he is an executive of the Victoria Emergency Physicians Association and the hospital Medical Staff Association, with special interests in patient education, information technology, mindfulness in medicine, business, and evidence-based happiness.

He works closely with the Divisions of Family Practice: Transitions in Care, with projects including Familiar Faces, which provides digital care plans for the most frequent users of local Emergency Departments.

A Mentor and Clinical Assistant Professor with the University of British Columbia Faculty of Medicine, he enjoys teaching and personal as well as professional development. He has presented at conferences and volunteered with community organizations such as the YMCA Camp Thunderbird and the Victoria Minor Hockey Association.

BULK SALES

Your company, institution, or organization may be interested in large volume purchases of this book for:

- Reselling
- Educational purposes
- Subscription and membership incentives
- Gifts and giveaways
- Fundraising campaigns

Discount schedule for bulk non-returnable sales

Volume	Savings	Shipping
11 - 20	20% Off plus TWO free copies	FREE
21 – 49	35% Off	FREE
50 - 200	50% Off	FREE
201 - 1000	62% Off	FREE
1000 +	Please contact for details	FREE

Excerpts, e-books, and e-excerpts also available.

Please contact me at book@drvoon.com.

CPSIA information can be obtained
at www.ICGtesting.com
Printed in the USA
LVHW040225080123
736411LV00003B/365

9 781777 603403